Gastroenterology Research and Clinical Developments

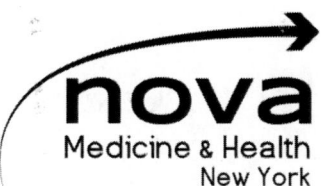

Gastroenterology Research and Clinical Developments

Effects of Healthful Bioactive Compounds on the Gastrointestinal Tract
Amir M. Mortazavian, PhD, Nasim Khorshidian, PhD, Zahra Yari, PhD
2022. ISBN: 978-1-68507-624-5 (Hardcover)
2022. ISBN: 978-1-68507-871-3 (eBook)

Probiotics and their Role in Health and Disease
Yusuf Olsen (Editor)
2021. ISBN: 978-1-53619-965-9 (Hardcover)
2021. ISBN: 978-1-53619-997-0 (eBook)

More information about this series can be found at
https://novapublishers.com/product-category/series/gastroenterology-research-and-clinical-developments/

Ujjwal Sonika

Gut Microbiome

Simplified! (For Medical, Nursing, Nutrition Students and Practitioners)

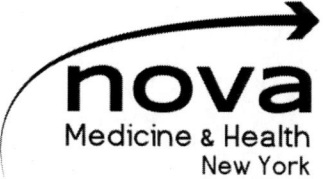

Copyright © 2022 by Nova Science Publishers, Inc.

https://doi.org/10.52305/GBKU2379

All rights reserved. No part of this book may be reproduced, stored in a retrieval system or transmitted in any form or by any means: electronic, electrostatic, magnetic, tape, mechanical photocopying, recording or otherwise without the written permission of the Publisher.

We have partnered with Copyright Clearance Center to make it easy for you to obtain permissions to reuse content from this publication. Simply navigate to this publication's page on Nova's website and locate the "Get Permission" button below the title description. This button is linked directly to the title's permission page on copyright.com. Alternatively, you can visit copyright.com and search by title, ISBN, or ISSN.

For further questions about using the service on copyright.com, please contact:
Copyright Clearance Center
Phone: +1-(978) 750-8400   Fax: +1-(978) 750-4470   E-mail: info@copyright.com

NOTICE TO THE READER

The Publisher has taken reasonable care in the preparation of this book, but makes no expressed or implied warranty of any kind and assumes no responsibility for any errors or omissions. No liability is assumed for incidental or consequential damages in connection with or arising out of information contained in this book. The Publisher shall not be liable for any special, consequential, or exemplary damages resulting, in whole or in part, from the readers' use of, or reliance upon, this material. Any parts of this book based on government reports are so indicated and copyright is claimed for those parts to the extent applicable to compilations of such works.

Independent verification should be sought for any data, advice or recommendations contained in this book. In addition, no responsibility is assumed by the Publisher for any injury and/or damage to persons or property arising from any methods, products, instructions, ideas or otherwise contained in this publication.

This publication is designed to provide accurate and authoritative information with regard to the subject matter covered herein. It is sold with the clear understanding that the Publisher is not engaged in rendering legal or any other professional services. If legal or any other expert assistance is required, the services of a competent person should be sought. FROM A DECLARATION OF PARTICIPANTS JOINTLY ADOPTED BY A COMMITTEE OF THE AMERICAN BAR ASSOCIATION AND A COMMITTEE OF PUBLISHERS.

Additional color graphics may be available in the e-book version of this book.

Library of Congress Cataloging-in-Publication Data

ISBN: 979-8-88697-340-2

Published by Nova Science Publishers, Inc. † New York

I loved reading this book and appreciate the way complex concepts are made extremely simple. A must-read for everyone who wants to understand the gut microbiome.

Vishal Sharma
Associate Professor, Gastroenterology
PGIMER, Chandigarh, India

An excellent book! Written from a healthcare professional's viewpoint.

Vipin Gupta
Consultant Gastroenterologist
North Bristol Trust, Bristol, UK

For Kanika and Oeshi

Contents

Preface xi

Acknowledgments xiii

Chapter 1   Gut Microbiota: Composition and Properties 1

Chapter 2   Gut Microbiota: Functions and Metabolites 17

Chapter 3   Role in Immune Development and Allergic Disorders 27

Chapter 4   Gut Microbiota: Role in Metabolic Diseases 33

Chapter 5   Gut Microbiota: Role in Cardiovascular Disease 45

Chapter 6   Role in Stress and Related Disorders 51

Chapter 7   Gut Microbiota: Role in Gastrointestinal Disorders 59

Chapter 8   The Microbiota Therapies 69

Bibliography 77

About the Author 99

Index 101

Preface

Health care professionals must know the basic concepts about gut microbiota. Gut microbiota has a huge impact on all the organ systems of the body. There has been exponential growth in the research on the gut microbiome and its clinical implications over the last few years. Besides gastrointestinal disorders, the role of microbiota is now established in obesity, metabolic diseases, neurological disease, cardiovascular diseases, genito-urinary diseases, and even skin disorders. This makes it necessary to know about the gut microbiome for all healthcare providers, including doctors, nurse practitioners, nutritionists, and students.

As the name suggests, this book teaches the concepts in a simple manner. The goal is to make you understand the basic terminologies in the field of the gut microbiome and teach about its functions and the factors which influence its composition. The various methods employed to study the microbiome are explained in easy terms so that the reader can grasp the complexities while studying a research article on gut microbiota in their field of expertise. The scientific studies on the gut microbiome are exploding in every area of health care, and this book aims to provide the armamentarium to enable the reader to navigate this vast sea of information effectively and purposefully.

The book's highlight is how it explores the pathophysiological mechanisms by which gut microbiota alterations contribute to the development of diseases. It provides a sound start based on which you can proceed with further learnings in your particular area of interest. The book provides a snapshot of the latest scientific literature and clinical applications of the gut microbiome in various illnesses such as diabetes, obesity, cardiovascular diseases, stress and anxiety, and gastrointestinal disorders, which will immediately bring immense value to your daily practice.

Although a considerable effort has been made to include the latest concepts, terminologies, and studies on the gut microbiome, the readers may find some concepts/terminologies missing or different from other texts or articles. This may either be due to the vastness of the available scientific literature and its tremendous pace of expansion or be purposefully omitted to maintain the simplicity of the text. I take full responsibility for such omissions/differences and shall be grateful if these be conveyed. I hope you find the book helpful and wish you good health and a healthy gut microbiome.

Ujjwal Sonika, MD, DM
Associate Professor, Gastroenterology, GB Pant Hospital,
Maulana Azad Medical College, New Delhi, India

26th July 2022

Acknowledgments

I thank my family for their continuous support and patience. This book is as much their effort as mine.

I am incredibly thankful to my colleagues for their constant motivation and encouragement while writing this book.

I sincerely thank all my esteemed teachers. It is their blessings that have made this work possible.

At last, my special thanks to Nova Publishers for their unwavering faith and for providing this fantastic opportunity to publish with them.

Chapter 1

Gut Microbiota: Composition and Properties

Goals

1. To know about the microorganisms present in gut microbiota.
2. To learn about factors having an impact on gut microbiota
3. To know the methods used to study gut microbiota
4. To understand various terminologies related to the gut microbiome

Gut Microbiota: Composition

A large number of microbes inhabit the human gastrointestinal (GI) tract and are collectively known as the gut microbiota. The skin, oral cavity, and vagina also harbor distinct microbes performing many essential functions. The gut microbiota, too, performs a range of functions necessary for our survival.

The terms microbiota and microbiome are subtly different. The combined gene pool of an organism is termed the genome. For example, all the genes present in our body constitute Human Genome. Similarly, the combined gene pool of all the microbes present in an ecosystem is termed the microbiome. Thus, the gut microbiome is the combined gene pool of microbes present in our gut. Or the gut microbiome is the total gene pool of the gut microbiota. The gut microbiota consists of all types of microbes, including bacteria, viruses, and fungi. The bacteria are the most well-studied among them, and their role in health and diseases is clearly described. The bacteria present in human intestines are hugely diverse. Around 10^{12} to $10^{14,}$ i.e., up to 100 trillion bacteria are present in our gut belonging to at least 1000 different species. Taxonomically, most of the gut bacteria belong to the four major phyla:

1. Firmicutes
2. Bacteroidetes
3. Proteobacteria
4. Actinobacteria

Firmicutes and Bacteroidetes are the most abundant, representing 90% of the bacteria in the gut microbiota. Firmicutes are Gram-positive bacteria. They are the prime fermenters of complex carbohydrates or dietary fiber. The most prominent Firmicute genera present in human intestines are Clostridium, Lactobacillus, Enterococcus, and Ruminicoccus.

Bacteroidetes are Gram-negative bacteria. They also ferment complex carbohydrates. Bacteroides, Prevotella, and Alistipes are the important genera belonging to this species.

Proteobacteria are present in smaller numbers in the healthy gut microbiota. Their increased abundance is associated with various diseases. They are gram-negative with an outer membrane that contains lipopolysaccharides (LPS). The first bacteria identified in the human intestines, Escherichia Coli, belongs to this phylum as well as many well-known pathogens such as Salmonella and Shigella.

Actinobacteria are gram-positive bacteria. The prime actinobacteria genus in the gut is Bifidobacterium. Though small in numbers, they are important members of healthy gut microbiota.

The majority of gut bacteria are anaerobes. They are 100–1000 times more than aerobic bacteria. They ferment the complex carbohydrates present in the diet. The human digestive enzymes do not break down complex carbohydrates. Their fermentation by the anaerobic gut bacteria leads to the production of different metabolites, the most important of which are short-chain fatty acids (SCFAs). These metabolites are a source of energy and play an important role in our metabolism, satiety signaling, and immune function.

Most of the gut bacteria reside in the colon or large intestine, approximately 10^9–10^{12} bacteria/ml followed by 10^4–10^8 bacteria/ml in the ileum and 10^1–10^3 bacteria/ml in the jejunum. The stomach usually contains few bacteria. The number of bacteria residing in the intestines of a single human is 1000 times the number of humans on earth.

We are more microbes than humans. The microbial cells in our body are ten times the human cells, and the microbial genes are 100 times more than the human genes. Before the Human Genome Project, which was completed in 2003, it was estimated that humans contain roughly 100,000 genes. However, the human genome has only 23000 genes, whereas 3.3 million microbial genes have already been found in the gut microbiome (Qin J et al. 2010). Recent estimates by scientists who gathered and analyzed all the publicly available DNA sequencing data on the human gut microbiome put this number at an astonishing 22 million genes (Braden et al. 2019). Lots of these microbial genes were shown to be unique to a single individual. Out of

22 million, 12.6 million microbial genes, i.e., more than 50%, were found only once and thus were unique to an individual. These microbial genes encode various proteins necessary for the survival of humans. The human genome doesn't encode these proteins, and thus we would not exist without the gut microbiota.

Gut Microbiota: Properties

The gut microbiota has a few inherent properties, which are:

1. *Stability:* The gut microbiota is stable in an individual. It starts developing soon after birth and changes rapidly during the initial years of life depending on weaning, exposure to different foods, and other environmental factors. At the start, the gut microbiota is simple and less diverse but becomes highly complex during early childhood. After that, during adult life, it remains relatively stable. There are many factors that influence the composition of gut microbiota. Still, if we study the gut bacterial composition of a healthy adult at different time points, a large proportion of gut bacteria remains the same.
2. *Plasticity:* Plasticity means that although the gut microbiota is stable, on this background of stability, there is a continuous change in its composition and metabolic behavior depending on the factors such as diet, exercise, use of medications, etc. For example, if someone includes more complex carbohydrates in their diet, the gut microbiota will respond and change. Similarly, the consumption of a high-fat diet will alter the gut microbiota in a different way. Thus, plasticity is the response of gut microbiota to an external factor.
3. *Resilience:* The gut microbiota is resilient. It has an inherent property to return to its original state. For example, the gut microbiota is altered when you take an antibiotic. But, after you stop, the gut microbiota reverts to its original composition over 4 to 6 weeks.

We can observe that these three properties are interrelated (Figure 1.1). The gut microbiota remains temporally stable but changes in response to external factors to variable degrees and tries to come back to its original composition when that factor is removed.

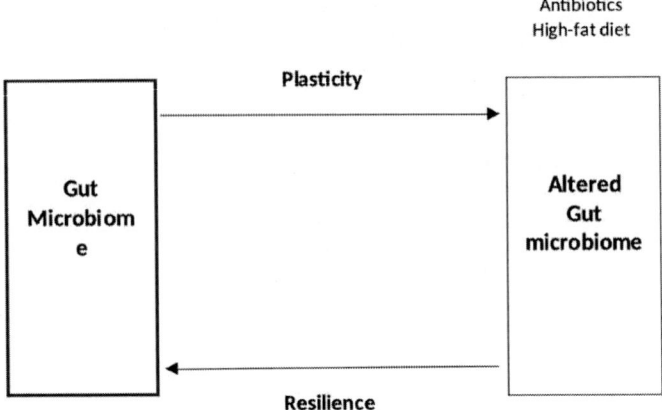

Figure 1.1. Plasticity and resilience of gut microbiota is plastic, i.e., its composition changes in response to factors such as antibiotics and a high-fat diet. But when it is removed, it reverts to it earlier state showing resilience.

These properties tell us that an effort to change the gut microbiota must be persistent. If you advise someone to improve their gut microbiota by dietary modification, lifestyle change, or probiotic supplements, it will need to be long-term and persistent. It means that adopting lifestyle measures that can be sustained life-long is better than expensive solutions such as probiotic supplements. However, short-term microbiota therapy is effective for diseases such as recurrent *Clostridium difficile* infection. The antibiotics-induced changes in the gut microbiota, which lead to *C. difficile* colitis, are temporary and can be mitigated by a single session of fecal microbiota transplant (FMT).

Factors Affecting the Gut Microbiota

The gut microbiota exists in a state of delicate balance. Various factors can alter its composition and functional capacity. Some factors such as diet are easily conceivable to have an impact on gut bacteria, but seemingly unrelated events like the mode of birth and growing up with an elder sibling or pets also have an effect. These factors are divided into two groups, modifiable and non-modifiable.

Non-Modifiable Factors

Genetics

Genes have a limited role in determining the composition and function of gut microbiota. Studies conducted on twins have revealed that although the initial gut microbiota is similar in twins, as they age, it becomes different, indicating a more significant role of the environmental factors.

Mode of Delivery

The mode of delivery has a profound impact on gut microbiota during the neonatal period. The fetal intestines were believed to be sterile. But recently, the fetal oral cavity and meconium have been found to have bacterial communities (Younge et al. 2019). The vaginal flora reaches the fetal intestines during the passage through the birth canal via the oral cavity. The vaginal flora during pregnancy is enriched with Lactobacillus, which gains access to the neonate's intestines and helps in digesting lactose, and helps in maintaining nutrition during infancy.

The babies born through cesarean section have an altered gut microbiota composition. Their gut is predominantly colonized with the bacteria present on the maternal skin rather than the vaginal flora (Dominguez-Bello et al. 2010). Their gut microbiota is less diverse, with a low abundance of Bacteroides, Bifidobacteria, and Lactobacillus. These differences are profound during the first three months of life and gradually disappear by the end of six months (Rutayisire et al. 2016). The higher incidence of asthma and allergic disorders in cesarean-born babies are shown to be due to these alterations in their gut microbiome (Gallazo et al. 2020).

Ethnicity

The gut bacteria differ among people of different countries and ethnicities. The gut microbiome of tribal populations is characterized by an abundance of bacteria that can digest complex plant carbohydrates. The Hadza people's gut microbiome, one of the last surviving hunter-gatherer tribes inhabiting the Eyasi Valley in northern Tanzania, is among the most diverse (Smits et al. 2017). Similarly, the gut microbiota of Americans is different from that of Indians and Indians from that of Chinese and Japanese (Dhakan et al. 2019). Most of these population-wise differences are due to different dietary habits, while genetics play a minor role.

Aging

The composition of the gut microbiome varies markedly with age. It is relatively simple at birth and becomes complex and diverse during early childhood. At the time of birth, we all have similar gut microbiota, the difference being only due to the mode of delivery. But as we age, the different environmental factors in the form of weaning and diet make the gut microbiota diverse. In a recent study, researchers analyzed the gut microbiota composition of infants at regular intervals till school age. The gut microbiota was similar up to three months of age and became gradually diverse till seven months. After seven months, there was a rapid increase in diversity. Bacteroidetes and Proteobacteria were present as early as one month of age, whereas Firmicutes arrived late. At school age, all the four major phyla were present. At 12 weeks, diet becomes the most crucial factor in the development of gut microbiota (Galazzo et al. 2020). From early childhood and during adult life, the gut microbiome remains complex and diverse. However, it again becomes less varied during old age. Proteobacteria also increase during old age (Xu et al. 2019).

Modifiable Factors

The modifiable factors have a more significant impact on the gut microbiota than the non-modifiable ones. These are:

Breast Feeding

Breast-fed infants have healthier and more diverse gut microbiota. They have a higher abundance of Bifidobacterium (Bezirtzoglou et al. 2011). Bifidobacteria utilizes the unique sugars in breast milk, called human milk oligosaccharides, which infants cannot digest themselves. Bifidobacteria are not present in the gut microbiota of formula-fed infants. They are vital members of the healthy gut microbiome. The infants also receive certain bacteria from the areola while sucking, which may contribute to the diversity of breast-fed infants' gut microbiota.

Diet

Diet is the most significant factor determining the composition and function of gut microbiota. The relationship between gut microbiota and diet is bidirectional, i.e., they both influence each other.

Among the dietary constituents, carbohydrates have the maximum impact on the gut microbiota. The carbohydrate digestion begins in the oral cavity by salivary amylase and is continued in the small intestine by pancreatic amylase and brush-border disaccharidases. However, many complex carbohydrates remain undigested. As noted earlier, they are fermented by the anaerobic bacteria present in the intestines. Dietary fiber is the source of complex carbohydrates and is found in unprocessed plant-based foods like whole grains, fruits, and vegetables. A high-fiber diet increases the gut bacterial diversity, and the abundance of Firmicutes, and reduces proteobacteria. (Simpson & Campbell 2015). The functional capacity of gut microbiota is altered even before the changes in gut microbial composition within two weeks after introducing a high-fiber diet (Barber et al. 2021). A high-fiber diet is beneficial in individuals with obesity and type 2 diabetes. Dietary supplementation with inulin, a complex carbohydrate, has been shown to improve insulin resistance in obese adults (Chambers et al. 2019). A recent meta-analysis of 9 RCTs on the role of dietary fiber in people with type 2 diabetes found that they increased the abundance of Bifidobacteria, raised SCFA levels, and reduced glycated hemoglobin compared to placebo (Ojo et al. 2020).

The impact of proteins on the gut microbiota is less pronounced and depends upon its source and composition. Plant-based proteins such as soy are associated with increased Lactobacillus and Bifidobacteria in the gut microbiota (Huang et al. 2016). Casein and whey are also found to be beneficial because of their high branched-chain amino acid content (Madsen et al. 2017). The sea-food proteins rich in taurine are associated with reduced proteobacteria and increased SCFA production in mice (Yu et al. 2016). A high protein diet in obese individuals increased gut bacterial diversity and raised Bifidobacteria and Akkermansia as compared to a regular protein diet (Dong et al. 2020).

The impact of fats on gut microbiota depends on both the quantity as well as the composition of the lipids. High-fat diet leads to reduced gut microbiome diversity and an increase in the proteobacteria. In a study conducted in China, researchers fed young, healthy individuals an iso-caloric diet with different fat quantities. Subjects were randomly assigned to receive a low fat (20% of energy through fats), moderate fat (30% of energy), and high fat (40% of energy) diet. They found that the high-fat diet group had reduced gut microbiota diversity. It highlighted that the effect of fat on the gut microbiome is independent of the total consumed calories. The short-chain fatty acids were also reduced in the high-fat diet group (Wan et al. 2019). The ratio of saturated fatty acids (SFA), mono-unsaturated fatty acids (MUFA), and polyunsaturated fatty acids (PUFA) in the diet are also shown to determine the gut microbiota composition. A diet high in MUFA and PUFA is associated with a higher

Bacteroidetes: Firmicutes ratio and increased lactic-acid bacteria (Costantini et al. 2017).

Polyphenols

Dietary polyphenols found in tea, fruits, vegetables, and cocoa are known to possess antioxidant properties and have an impact on the gut microbiota. They are compounds with diverse chemical compositions such as flavonols, flavones, phenolic acids, and anthocyanin. The dietary intake of polyphenols is associated with increased Bifidobacterium and Lactobacillus, having a beneficial impact on the human gut microbiota (Ma and Chen 2020).

Fermented Foods

Fermented foods are an excellent dietary source of beneficial microbes. Humankind has been fermenting food for centuries to increase its shelf life and nutritional value. Common examples of fermented foods include curd, yogurt, Miso, Sauerkraut, Kanji, and Kimchi. The fermentation process utilizes microbes to break down the complex sugars present in food, similar to what gut bacteria do in the intestines. Fermented foods are shown to alter the human gut microbiome composition in beneficial ways. In a recent trial, a 10-week fermented food rich diet led to increased gut bacterial diversity and decreased pro-inflammatory markers (Wastyk HC et al. 2021). A large meta-analysis showed that fermented dairy foods, especially yogurt, reduce the risk of diabetes in humans (Zhang K, Pai B & Deng Z. 2021).

Dietary Patterns

The Western diet includes high intakes of red meat, pre-packaged processed foods, refined grains, corn (and high-fructose corn syrup), and low intakes of fruits, vegetables, whole grains, fish, nuts, and seeds. It is rich in saturated fats and refined sugars and poor in unsaturated fats and fiber. In a Korean study, researchers compared the gut microbiota of individuals on the western diet for four weeks. They then crossed over to the traditional Korean diet, rich in fish, fiber, and fermented foods. They found that after the 4-week western diet, the gut bacteria diversity decreased, which subsequently increased after the Korean diet (Shin et al. 2019). The bacterium Weissella was increased on the Korean diet. Weissella is a probiotic bacterium that ferments Kimchi, a fermented vegetable dish widely consumed in Korea (Jung et al. 2011). The fact that the 4-week western diet altered the gut microbiota in Korean individuals highlights that diet has a greater impact on gut microbiome than ethnicity.

The Mediterranean diet reduces the incidence of coronary artery disease (Kromhout et al. 1995). It was first defined by Ancel Keys as being low in saturated fat and high in vegetable oils, particularly olive oil, and is consumed in Mediterranean countries. It is high in vegetables, fruits, nuts, fish, and unsaturated fats, with a low intake of red meat, saturated fats, and dairy foods. Studies have shown that adherence to the Mediterranean diet increases the abundance of Firmicutes and Bifidobacteria in the gut microbiome and leads to increased production of short-chain fatty acids (SCFAs) (De Filippis et al. 2016) (Mitsou et al. 2017).

Enterotypes

The gut microbiota is traditionally divided into two distinct enterotypes based on bacterial composition. Enterotype 1 is characterized by the abundance of Bacteroides. It is associated with a diet rich in animal protein and fat, whereas enterotype 2 is associated with a carbohydrate-rich diet and is abundant in Prevotella (Arumugum et al. 2011). The enterotype-based classification is not used much in clinical studies. The alterations in gut microbiota associated with a disease are not characterized by changes in enterotypes. They are usually at the level of genus or species.

Exercise

Exercise has a strong and independent effect on the gut microbiota irrespective of diet and Body Mass Index (BMI). It was first noted in 2008 in a Japanese study. The study compared the gut microbiota of sedentary (non-exercised) and exercised mice (Matsumoto et al. 2008). The exercised group was placed in cages with wheels with a design that forced mice to use them. The microbiota of the exercised mice showed increased production of SCFAs.

The beneficial effects of exercise on gut microbiota composition and function are also shown in humans. A study conducted on international rugby players in Ireland compared their gut microbiome with healthy Irish adults. The gut microbiome of the rugby players was found to be more diverse. In particular, there was greater diversity among the Firmicutes in the gut microbiota of rugby players as compared to the healthy adults (Clarke et al. 2014). In another study, Estaki et al. (2016) analyzed the fecal microbiota of 39 individuals with different fitness levels but comparable diets. Peak oxygen uptake (VO_2 max, also known as maximal oxygen consumption, maximal oxygen uptake, or maximal aerobic capacity) is a gold standard indicator of cardio-respiratory fitness and endurance. A high VO_2 max indicates better cardio-respiratory fitness. The study found that regardless of the diet, cardiorespiratory fitness correlated with increased gut microbial diversity and abundance of butyrate-producing bacteria, such as Clostridiales and Lachnospiraceae (Estaki et al. 2016). Exercise is also shown to reduce the proteobacteria in the gut microbiota. These beneficial changes in the gut microbiota are observed as early as six weeks after beginning the exercise (Allen et al. 2018).

Sleep

Sleep affects the gut microbiota. Inadequate sleep leads to harmful changes in the gut microbiota. As little as two days of sleep deprivation can alter the gut microbiota composition leading to decreased insulin sensitivity and an increased propensity to develop diabetes (Benedict et al. 2016). Getting fragmented sleep or sleeping at unnatural times can also alter the gut microbiome. A study on mice revealed that just four weeks of altered sleep cycle reduces the gut microbial diversity (Deaver et al. 2018).

Antibiotics

Of all the medications, antibiotics have the highest impact on gut microbiota. Antibiotics do not differentiate between the commensal gut bacteria and pathogens. The consumption of antibiotics decreases the number as well as the diversity of gut bacteria within 3–4 days. After one week of discontinuing antibiotics, gut microbiota begins to recover and achieves composition similar to the pre-antibiotic period in one month. However, it takes more than six months for it to recover fully. Loss of commensal bacteria due to antibiotics provides an opportunity for pathogens to grow, leading to gastrointestinal infections. One such example is *Clostridium difficile* infection, which typically occurs in the setting of antibiotic use. The incidence of *C. difficile* colitis is rising across the globe due to the increased use of antibiotics.

Other Medications

A large number of medicines alter the gut microbiota. In an extensive study investigating the impact of drugs on the gut microbiota, out of 835 non-antibiotic medicines, 200 restricted the growth of at least one type of bacteria, and around 5% of medicines affected at least ten types of bacteria (Maier et al. 2018). Some commonly used medications which alter gut microbiota are anti-inflammatory drugs, antipsychotics, cancer chemotherapy, proton-pump inhibitors, and metformin. Most of these decrease the diversity of the gut microbiota.

The anti-inflammatory drugs and proton-pump inhibitors (PPI) are amongst the most commonly used prescription and over-the-counter medications. PPIs inhibit acid secretion in the stomach. They are widely consumed to treat acidity, bloating, and heartburn. In a study, the stool samples of the participants using PPI showed a reduction in the gut microbiota diversity. PPI consumption altered 20 % of the bacterial species present in the intestines (Imhann et al. 2016). Furthermore, PPIs increase the presence of oral bacteria in the intestines. As the oral bacteria pass into the stomach along with the ingested food, they are killed by the acid present in the stomach. However, as the acid secretion is suppressed upon PPI consumption, these bacteria reach the intestine. The increased oral bacteria in the intestines is associated with poor outcomes in patients with liver cirrhosis.

The non-steroidal anti-inflammatory drugs (NSAIDs) also reduce bacterial diversity and increase the number of potential enteric pathogens in the gut microbiota (Rogers and Aronoff 2016). The effect of medications on gut microbiota may also be beneficial. Metformin, the most commonly used medicine for the treatment of diabetes, alters the gut microbiome leading to increased short-chain fatty acid production, which may contribute to its therapeutic effect (Wu et al. 2017).

To conclude, the most important determinants of gut microbiota composition and function are modifiable. They include breastfeeding and lifestyle measures such as diet, exercise, and sleep.

Methods to Study Gut Microbiome

The rapid progress in the methods to study biological systems forms the basis of gut microbiome research. Traditionally, the bacteria are grown on culture media which is a huge limitation in studying gut bacteria because of their large numbers and fastidious nutrition requirements. They would compete with each other, and it would be impossible to identify the grown species.

The advent of DNA sequencing invented to study the human genome has led to the development of a novel way to identify non-cultivable bacteria. These sequencing methods identify the genes expressed by the gut microbiota and can also tell its functions. Finally, the advancements in mass spectroscopy and NMR spectroscopy have made it possible to identify the metabolites produced by the bacteria, which are the final microbial products, and help understand the mechanisms by which the gut microbiota shape our health.

(Metabolome is the complete set of metabolites found in a biological sample) (Figure 1.2).

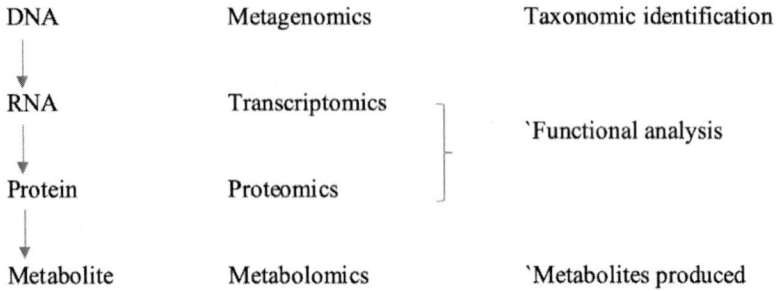

Figure 1.2. Central dogma and the equivalent study of the gut microbiota.

Table 1.1. Comparisons of methods to study gut bacteria

	Conventional Methods	**New Methods**
Growth and Identification of Specie	Culture media	16 S rRNA gene sequencing
Enzymes	Chemical reactions	Transcriptomics/Proteomics
Metabolites	None	Metabolomics

Identification of Species

The gut microbiome has a large number of microbial species. There are more than 1000 bacterial species present in the intestines. How are they identified?

Each bacterial cell has 16 S ribosomal RNA, which is part of the ribosome. The 16S RNA gene is highly conserved across bacterial species, but it also has a hypervariable region that is unique and helps in the identification of bacteria. Thus, the 16S ribosomal RNA gene forms the basis of the techniques used to identify the bacteria in a biological sample.

The first step in the metagenomic analysis of stool samples is the extraction of nucleic acid. Following this, the PCR amplification of species-specific 1500 base pairs long 16S ribosomal RNA genes is done. PCR-based amplification is carried out by using universal and specific primers. The 16S rRNA gene amplicons which PCR generates are then sequenced, and bacterial species are identified. Next-Generation Sequencing (NGS), which is fast and cheap, has revolutionized DNA sequencing and is now commonly used for microbiome analysis. There are many other culture-independent methods used to identify bacterial species, and all of them rely on the 16S rRNA gene.

Function Analysis

After identifying the bacteria present in the gut microbiota, the next logical step is to know what these bacteria are doing. This knowledge can help better understand their role in our health and various diseases.

The NGS plays a significant role in this too. As the NGS method is fast, the whole genome can be sequenced in a relatively short time. While the 16S rRNA gene sequencing identifies the bacterial specie, the whole genome sequencing identifies all the genes in a given sample and thus tells about the function of gut microbiota. NGS can also sequence RNA, which has the advantage of identifying only those genes that are expressed in the given sample. The complete RNA content of a sample is known as transcriptome. However, it is more expensive and requires greater technical expertise.

Metabolites

Studying metabolites produced by gut microbiota is the final step in understanding its role. Mass spectroscopy and NMR spectroscopy can detect and identify all the metabolites present in a sample. This method of studying the metabolites is called metabolomics. However, the technologies used for metabolomics are not widely available and are very expensive.

Most of the scientific studies analyzing the role of gut microbiota primarily look into the number and diversity of bacteria using the 16S rRNA gene amplification. Many of them also identify a group of species or a particular specie associated with the disease in question. Very few studies look into functional analysis and metabolomics as they are expensive and not widely available.

Gut Virome

The gut microbiota consists of not only bacteria but also fungi and viruses. We will discuss each of them briefly.

The complete gut viral community or the gut virome is highly diverse, like the gut bacterial community. The gut viruses are predominantly bacteriophages, which are the viruses that infect bacteria. They are mainly DNA viruses. Phages are the most abundant form of life on earth and outnumber bacteria by 10:1 in most habitats. However, in the human gut, phages are believed to exist at levels comparable to their bacterial hosts (Kim et al. 2011). As bacteriophages are its prime constituents, gut virome acts mainly through its effects on the bacteria present in our intestines.

There are three ways bacteriophages can affect gut microbial composition and function.

1. They can lyse and kill the host bacteria and thus influence the bacterial community's structure.
2. They can transfer genes between the bacteria by the process of transduction and can influence their function.
3. They can provide genetic information to the bacterial host cell and influence their function.

The human gut virome composition, just like the bacteria, is characterized by a high degree of inter-personal variation and temporal stability. Studies have reported retention of >95% of viral genotypes within one individual over one year (Reyes et al. 2010) and 80 % of genotypes over 2.5 years (Minot et al. 2012). The individuals consuming similar diets tend to have identical gut viromes (Wu et al. 2011).

The gut virome is identified to perform a wide range of functions. Recent metagenomic studies have revealed that gut-associated phages encode genes that are generally beneficial for intestinal bacteria, including functions that help host bacteria adapt to their environment and help maintain host-microbiome stability. For example, analysis of the gut virome in mice revealed that following exposure to antibiotics, gut phage populations were enriched for genes associated with antibiotic resistance and those related to gut colonization (Modi et al. 2013).

Recently, the gut virome has been shown to have a role in human health and diseases. The obese individuals have reduced gut virome diversity compared to the lean individuals. The gut virome changes were more pronounced in obese individuals with type 2 diabetes (Yang et al. 2021). Gut virome transplantation has been done in mice and shown to be successful (Rasmussen et al. 2020). The role of gut phages is also being studied in several other diseases and further research will clarify their clinical and therapeutic implications.

Gut Mycobiome

Gut mycobiome is all the fungi present in the human intestines. Similar to gut viruses, there is a recent surge in the knowledge about gut fungi and their role in various diseases.

The human gut mycobiome is diverse, though less than the gut bacteriome. The most common fungal genera found in human fecal samples are Saccharomyces, Malassezia, Candida, Cyberlindnera, Penicillium, Cladosporium, and Aspergillus (Nash AK et al. 2017). The fungal genera in human samples are identified and taxonomically classified by 18 S rRNA and ITS-2 gene sequencing. Out of the 15 most common fungal genera, 8 are yeasts. The gut fungi also live attached to the intestinal mucosa, and the gut mucosal mycobiome is different and more stable than the fecal mycobiome.

The fungi colonize the human gut during childbirth, similar to the bacteria. The gut mycobiome of vaginally born newborns has more Candida, whereas caesarean-born babies have more Malassezia found on the maternal skin (Azevedo MJ et al. 2020). It becomes more diverse during infancy, especially with the initiation of breastfeeding. Contrary to bacteria, the diversity of gut fungi reduces after infancy. Young adults have less diverse gut mycobiome than infants, and the diversity is further reduced in the elderly. Diet is a major determinant of the gut mycobiome composition in adult life.

The role of gut mycobiome is increasingly recognized in various diseases. The inflammatory bowel disease, both Ulcerative colitis and Crohn's disease, show increased fungal diversity and alteration in the gut mycobiome composition. The gut mycobiome composition is also altered in colorectal cancers (Coker OO et al. 2019) and metabolic disorders such as diabetes (Jayasudha R et al. 2020). Recently, a fungus used in the packaged food industry was found abundantly in the diseased intestinal mucosal samples of patients with Crohn's disease (Jain U et al. 2021). This fungus Debaryomyces hansenii is used for surface ripening of cheese and meat products. Whether these gut mycobiome changes are simply associations or have a causal relationship is not yet clear. Future studies will provide more causal and therapeutic evidence for the use of fungi in human diseases.

Chapter 2

Gut Microbiota: Functions and Metabolites

Goals

1. To know about the functions performed by gut microbiota in humans
2. To understand the concept of the gut barrier and intestinal permeability
3. To know about the gut microbiota metabolites

Gut Microbiota: Functions

The bacteria were established as human pathogens in 1854 A.D with the discovery of Vibrio cholerae in the small intestine of patients who died of cholera. In 1885, the discovery of E. coli in the stools of children by Theodor Escherich showed that bacteria also exist as commensals in human intestines. But they were not believed to perform any important function. Later, the gut bacteria were discovered to synthesize a few vitamins. However, in the last 15 years, with the advent of newer techniques of metagenomics and metabolomics, it is proven that gut bacteria perform many vital functions that are essential for our survival.

Energy Absorption

The gut microbiome helps in energy absorption as they ferment the indigestible carbohydrates from our diet and thus 'unlock' the calories which otherwise would have been wasted. Experiments in mice have revealed that we need gut bacteria for optimum absorption of calories. In a study, the germ-free mice were compared with the conventionally raised mice for their weight and feeding patterns. At similar calorie intake, the weight of the germ-free mice was found to be significantly less than that of the wild-type mice (Bäckhed et al. 2004).

Fermentation of Complex Carbohydrates

The Firmicutes and the Bacteroidetes are the major phyla that ferment complex polysaccharides into absorbable simpler compounds. For e.g., *Bacteroides thetaiotaomicron* produces enzymes that break down complex O-glycan mucins, which are otherwise non-digestible, into absorbable carbohydrates (Martens et al. 2008). It is estimated that complex carbohydrates contribute 10%-30% of the total energy provided by the food, which is un-absorbable without gut bacteria.

The gut microbiota does not utilize all complex carbohydrates. Only a few of them are digested by the microbial enzymes and are known as Microbiota Accessible Carbohydrates or MACs. Thus, not all complex carbohydrates are MACs. MACs themselves are not a fixed entity of a particular set of carbohydrates. Depending upon the gut microbial composition, they differ among populations, individuals, and even within a single individual. Let's say population A has a particular bacterium X in their gut microbiota which ferments a specific complex carbohydrate Y, and population B does not have the bacterium X. Then Y is a MAC for population A but not for B. One such example is porphyran, a complex carbohydrate present in the marine red alga. It is a MAC for the Japanese population as their gut bacteria can metabolize it. However, the same porphyran is not a MAC for North Americans or Europeans. The Japanese gut microbiota metabolizes porphyran because their diet contains abundant porphyran in marine seaweed, while the western population does not consume it regularly. This highlights a dynamic and reciprocal relationship between gut microbiota and diet, which incidentally is the most critical factor influencing gut microbiome composition.

Dietary fibers are of many types, including resistant starch, cellulose, hemicellulose, guar gum, galactooligosaccharides, fructooligosaccharides, and inulin. Several microbial enzymes are required to digest a single kind of dietary fiber usually produced by different bacterial species. Thus, a host must harbor all the necessary bacteria to derive maximum benefit. The prime species responsible for the fermentation of a specific fiber is termed a keystone species. For example, Ruminococcus bromii is a keystone species in the fermentation of resistant starch (Ze et al. 2012). The final product or metabolites of fermentation of dietary fibers are, thus, a result of the symbiotic relationship between several gut bacteria.

Maintaining the Intestinal Barrier

The gut or intestinal barrier is comprised of epithelial cells, intercellular junctions, and the mucous layer. The epithelial cells adhere closely to each other with the help of intercellular junctions (ICJ). There are various types of ICJ, e.g., tight junctions, adherens junctions, gap junctions, and desmosomes. The tight junctions are the strongest and keep the epithelial cells bound to each other. Claudins and Occludins are the proteins that form tight junctions.

Although the epithelial cells closely adhere to each other, there is a space between them known as the paracellular space. The bacteria and various molecules can pass through the paracellular space and reach the blood vessels or the lymphatics. This property of the intestines to allow specific molecules/particles/bacteria to pass through is termed intestinal permeability or *gut permeability*. Gut permeability isn't a rigid entity. It changes in response to different stimuli. For example, alcohol increases intestinal permeability. It is also increased in various diseases such as cirrhosis, acute pancreatitis, celiac disease, and inflammatory bowel diseases. The term 'leaky gut' is also used to denote the increased gut permeability. When the gut permeability increases, many undesirable substances can pass through, resulting in illness. A typical example is the development of spontaneous bacterial peritonitis (SBP), an infection of ascitic fluid in patients with cirrhosis. Increased intestinal permeability in cirrhotic individuals allows the translocation of bacteria, primarily E. coli, into the ascitic fluid leading to SBP.

The gut bacteria help in maintaining the intestinal barrier function in several ways. The most important being the production of short-chain fatty acid, butyrate. Butyrate is the source of energy for the intestinal epithelial cells and is required to keep them healthy. Healthy epithelial cells keep the gut barrier intact. Butyrate also improves the gut barrier by increasing the tight junction assembly, leading to strong intercellular junctions (Peng et al. 2009). It also increases intestinal mucous production and thus thickens the mucous layer, the third component of the gut barrier (Shimotoyodome et al. 2000).

The bacteria also interact with the intestinal epithelial cells and promote their proliferation, which contributes to healing the gut barrier after an injury. (Thomas et al. 2018). The lifestyle diseases such as diabetes are characterized by the presence of persistent low-grade inflammation. The pro-inflammatory molecules gain entry into the circulation through our gut. An inefficient gut barrier leads to the increased entry of such molecules into the systemic circulation. The gut microbiota help reduce these inflammatory molecules by keeping the gut barrier intact.

Development and Maintenance of Immunity

The immune system protects us from infections. Let us briefly overview the working of the immune system to understand the role of gut microbiota in its development. Our immune system works in two steps. The first step is the identification of infectious agents. And the second step is their elimination.

The immune system has a remarkable capability to distinguish self-antigen from non-self antigens, which forms the basis of the first step of identifying pathogens. A molecule that activates the immune system is termed an *antigen*. It can be a protein, a polysaccharide, or a combination of the two. Self-antigens are our own antigens that the immune system recognizes as harmless, and hence, it doesn't mount a response against them under normal conditions. The non-self antigens are those that come from the external environment. The various pathogens and their molecules are non-self antigens. These are identified and eliminated by the immune system to prevent infections. But, we also encounter many non-self antigens that are not harmful to us. We inhale many external substances, such as pollen grains, dust particles, and pollutants. Another even bigger portal of entry for non-self-antigens into our body is the gut. We eat food that has molecules that are not intrinsic to our bodies. However, our immune system does not mount a response against them. Similarly, a large number of bacteria also reside in our intestines without an immune response. This property of the immune system of not mounting a response to an antigen is termed *tolerance*.

The immune system has two components- innate and acquired. The innate immune cells identify the microbes by specific patterns not present on human cells. Such patterns are called Pathogen Associated Molecular Patterns (PAMPs). They are recognized by pattern recognition receptors of immune cells (mainly dendritic cells), following which an immune response is generated. The adaptive immune system identifies the external antigens by displaying them on the antigen presenting cells (APC). The APCs present the antigens to the T-helper cells, which, based on the type of antigens, mount either an antibody-producing B-cell response producing antibodies or cytotoxic T-cell response. Both ultimately eliminate the pathogens.

The immune cells reside in specialized tissues such as lymph nodes, spleen, and thymus, which together form the structural framework of the immune system. But a large number of immune cells are also present in our intestines. In fact, the gut is the largest immune organ of the human body.

So what happens in the gut immune system that, even when it recognizes non-self antigens, does not mount a response against them? The cells and antibodies comprising the gut immune system respond differently to the external antigens. When an external antigen is presented by the APCs in the gut, it stimulates regulatory T cells (Tregs), which suppress the further activation of the immune cascade. *Lactobacillus reuteri* and *Lactobacillus casei* in gut microbiota lead to increased production of Tregs and thus help in the proper functioning of the gut immune system (Smits et al. 2005). *Bifidobacterium infantis* has also been shown to increase the Tregs in healthy human volunteers (Konieczna et al. 2012). Thus, the gut microbiota helps in the development of tolerance in the gut immune system.

The gut immune system also needs to identify harmful pathogens and eliminate them. The gut bacteria play an essential role in developing the gut immune system by providing antigenic stimulation to the immune cells during infancy and early childhood (Dzidic et al. 2018). They train the immune system, which is essential as it has been shown that germ-free mice are more susceptible to infection by intestinal pathogens than normal mice. As a newborn, we are protected from infections by maternal antibodies. Our own immune system is naïve. The gut microbiota educates the immune system. When germ-free mice are provided with bacterial flora, they develop more diverse immune cells and a robust immune system.

Protection from Pathogenic Bacteria

The gut microbiota actively blocks the growth of pathogens. Both the commensals and the pathogenic bacteria require nutrients to grow and multiply. They compete with each other for nutrients and space. Reduction in good gut bacteria due to poor diet, disease, or antibiotics allows the gut to be available to the pathogens. *Clostridium difficile* colitis is the prime example of such an infection. It occurs in patients with recent oral antibiotic use. Antibiotics do not differentiate between the pathogens and the commensals and kill both. The alteration of the gut microbiome allows the germination of *C. difficile* spores, which otherwise would not have germinated in healthy individuals. *C. difficile* infection is treated with antibiotics, metronidazole, and vancomycin. But the recurrence rate is high. Fecal microbial transplant (FMT) from a healthy donor is the treatment of choice for recurrent *C. difficile* infection. The engraftment of bacteria from the donor stools into the recipient's intestines leads to the normalization of gut microbiota and prevents further recurrence. Recurrent *C. difficile* infection is the first clinical condition for which FMT is recommended. The gut microbiota also fights the pathogens directly by producing substances that kill other bacteria, called bacteriocins.

Vitamin Synthesis

Thiamine, folate, biotin, riboflavin, and pantothenic acid are water-soluble vitamins synthesized by the gut microbiota. Vitamin K, a fat-soluble vitamin, is also produced by gut bacteria.

Gut Microbiota Metabolites

Gut bacteria produce a wide variety of substances by fermentation of complex carbohydrates and enzymatic actions on amino acids and bile acids. These substances perform a range of functions and are termed Gut Microbiota Metabolites (GMMs). The carbohydrate and amino-acid pathways producing GMMs are called the saccharolytic and proteolytic pathways respectively. GMMs can either be exclusively produced by the gut microbiota like Short Chain Fatty Acids (SCFAs), or they can be made by human cells as well, e.g., Succinate and Serotonin (Figure 2.1).

GMMs act via multiple mechanisms:

1. *Endocrine*: Serotonin is a hormone produced both by endocrine cells as well as bacteria in the intestines. It enters the bloodstream and acts on the central nervous system.
2. *Paracrine*: Both Serotonin and SCFAs act on other cells within the intestines. Serotonin act via HT receptors and influence gut motility. Butyrate, an SCFA, acts on L-cells to produce Peptide YY.
3. *Genetic*: Acetate, an SCFA act at the genetic level in the immune cells.
4. *Direct*: Butyrate is a source of energy for the colonic epithelial cells and thus provides nourishment.
5. *Immune function*: GMMs have anti-inflammatory properties. Acetate induces the Foxp3 expression leading to the generation of the T regs phenotype that alleviates the immune reaction.

Although a large number of GMMs are produced by gut microbiota, let us learn about a few in detail as they play a key role in our health.

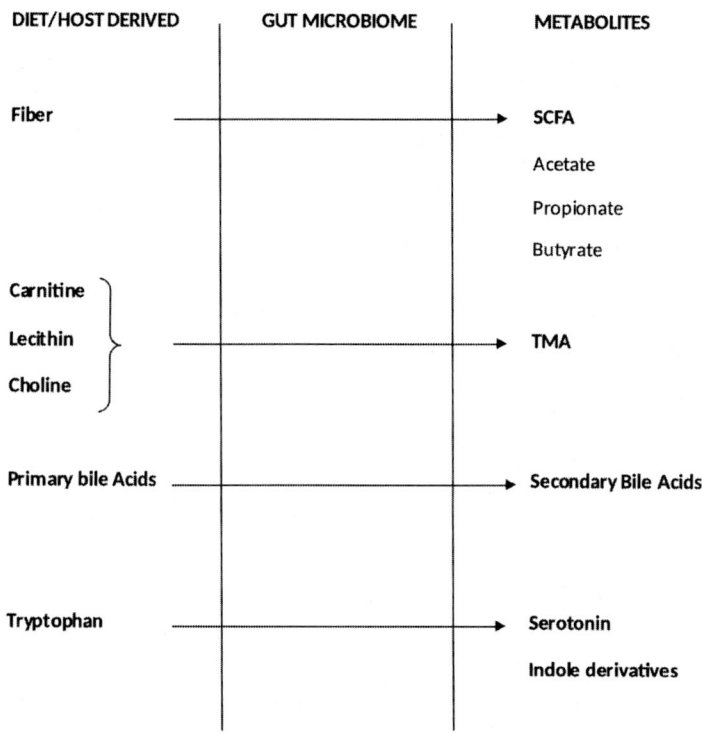

Figure 2.1. Schematic diagram showing the microbial transformation of dietary or host-derived substances leading to the generation of gut microbiota metabolites.

Short Chain Fatty Acids

Short-chain fatty acids (SCFA) are an essential class of compounds. Fats, along with carbohydrates and proteins, are the primary macronutrients. Saturated fats are solid at room temperature. They include all the animal fats like butter, ghee, the fat present in red meat, and coconut oil. The unsaturated fats are liquid at room temperature. They include all the fats of plant origin except coconut oil and fish oils. There are a few fats that are not produced in our bodies. They are termed essential fatty acids. All the essential fatty acids are unsaturated fats. The fats are classified based on the number of carbon atoms present in them. The fats with 2, 3, and 4 carbon atoms are termed short-chain, from 6 to 12 carbon atoms as medium-chain and more than 12 as long-chain fatty acids. Thus, acetate, propionate, and butyrate are SCFAs containing 2, 3, and 4 carbon atoms, respectively.

SCFA, like essential fatty acids, cannot be synthesized by human cells. Instead, they are produced by the microbial fermentation of complex carbohydrates in the intestines. Bacteroidetes mainly produce acetate and propionate, while Firmicutes mostly produce butyrate. SCFA are also present in the diet, and as saturated fats are usually present in animal fats, SCFs are also present in them. Butter, which derives its name from butyric acid, is a source of SCFAs. The complex chemical reactions and microbial enzymes involved in the generation of SCFAs are well elucidated but are beyond the scope of this book. SCFAs perform many functions and are the most important metabolite produced by the gut microbiota.

The SCFAs are the predominant source of energy for the colocytes, the cells that absorb water and maintain hydration. The volume of the ileal effluent reaching the caecum is 1.5 to 2 liters, while the stool volume of a healthy adult is only 200 ml per day. The water absorption in the colon occurs by osmosis. The sodium ion is actively absorbed in the colon via sodium channels, leading to the generation of an osmotic gradient across the colonic epithelium, which causes the absorption of water from the lumen. Sodium absorption is an energy-dependent process as it occurs against the concentration gradient, which is provided by the SCFAs.

Butyrate plays a vital role in satiety signaling. It acts on L-cells in the ileum, releasing Peptide YY. Peptide YY is a hormone. It reaches the brain via circulation and provides the satiety signal. In studies conducted on mice, long-term oral butyrate supplementation has been shown to reduce total food intake and prevent obesity and diabetes (Li et al. 2018). Butyrate reduces intestinal inflammation and colonic epithelial injury. Thus, it prevents colon cancer, as longstanding epithelial injury can ultimately lead to colon cancer (Hamer et al. 2008).

Propionate, another SCFA, is absorbed from the intestines and reaches the liver, where it promotes fatty acid oxidation and prevents fatty liver.

Acetate, the most abundant SCFA, acts at the genetic level (Zeng and Chi 2015). It induces Foxp3 expression in T-cells and has been shown to reduce asthma and allergy in mice. Infants who lack the acetate-producing gut bacteria are more likely to develop allergic diseases during childhood (Galazzo et al. 2020).

Methylamines

Trimethylamine (TMA) is an amine synthesized by the microbial enzymes from dietary components; L-carnitine, lecithin, choline, and betaine. They are present in various food sources such as red meat, fish, eggs, and dairy products. TMA is absorbed in the intestines and reaches the liver via the portal circulation, where it is oxidized into trimethylamine-N-oxide (TMAO), predominantly by the enzyme monooxygenase 3.

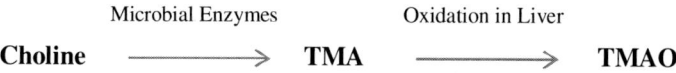

Choline $\xrightarrow{\text{Microbial Enzymes}}$ **TMA** $\xrightarrow{\text{Oxidation in Liver}}$ **TMAO**

TMAO levels are shown to correlate with cardiovascular diseases in humans. TMAO increases platelet activity and the formation of foam cells within atherosclerotic plaques. It can lead to an increased risk of atherosclerosis progression and thrombus formation. It also induces multiple inflammatory proteins, such as interleukin 6, cyclooxygenase 2, E-selectin, and intercellular adhesion molecule 1.

A study of more than 4000 patients undergoing coronary angiography found that, after adjustment for all major risk factors, the rate of major adverse cardiovascular events was significantly higher (adjusted hazard ratio about 1.5) among patients with the highest blood levels of TMAO compared to those with the lowest (Tang WH et al. 2013). A systematic review including 19 prospective studies found that high levels of TMAO and TMAO precursors (L-carnitine, choline, or betaine) were associated with significantly increased risk for major adverse cardiovascular events. (Heianza et al. 2017).

Secondary Bile Acids

Both the SCFAs and TMA are derived from the microbial action on dietary substances. In contrast, secondary bile acids are generated from the host-derived compounds' primary bile acids. The role of secondary bile acids is discussed in chapter 4.

Tryptophan Metabolites

The amino acid Tryptophan is metabolized by the gut microbial enzymes into many different metabolites. The most important of them are Serotonin and Indole derivatives.

Serotonin acts as a neurotransmitter and hormone. It is known as the Happy hormone. It plays a wide variety of roles in the GI tract as well as the central nervous system. Its functions are discussed in detail in chapter 6.

Tryptophan is also metabolized to indole by the microbial enzyme tryptophanase. Various bacteria species express different types of tryptophanase, leading to the production of a range of indole derivatives, e.g., indole-3-pyruvate, indole-3-aldehyde, indole-3-acetic acid, indole-3-lactic acid, indole-3-propionic acid, and others.

Indole derivatives perform several beneficial functions in humans. These include:

1. Indole derivatives act on immune cells in the intestines via a receptor called aryl hydrocarbon receptor (AhR) (Qiu et al. 2012). They exert an anti-inflammatory action through this interaction.
2. They help in maintaining the integrity of the intestinal barrier by increasing the expression of epithelial tight junctions and increasing mucous production from the goblet cells (Shimada et al. 2013).
3. Indole increases the secretion of GLP-1 from the enteroendocrine L-cells and thus plays a role in blood glucose control and satiety signaling (Chimeral et al. 2014).

Indole derivatives play an essential role in liver diseases. In a study on non-alcoholic fatty liver disease (NAFLD), the serum indole levels were lower in obese individuals compared to lean. Serum indole also correlated inversely with liver fat content. When mice were fed a high-fat diet with indole, the increase in liver fat content and inflammation was much less than when the high-fat diet was given alone (Ma et al. 2020).

To conclude, gut microbiota performs many of its functions through GMMs. Alterations in the GMM levels, such as butyrate and indole derivatives, are associated with various diseases. They have considerable therapeutic potential, which may be realized in the near future.

Chapter 3

Role in Immune Development and Allergic Disorders

Goals

1. To know briefly about the gut immune system and its differences in neonates and adults
2. To know about the role of the microbiota in the development of the gut immune system
3. Understanding the Hygiene hypothesis
4. To know the relevant clinical implications

The gastrointestinal tract (GIT) is the largest immune organ in the human body. It encounters a large number of antigens. The gut immune cells are present in the epithelium as intra-epithelial lymphocytes and in lamina propria, which contains dendritic cells, lymphocytes, and plasma cells. Besides, organized lymphoid follicles called Peyer's patches are present in submucosa. All these, together, form mucosa-associated lymphoid tissue or MALT, which denotes the immune cells present in relation to the mucosa of organs such as GIT or respiratory tract. The MALT in the GIT is termed GALT, gut-associated lymphoid tissue.

The immune system is not the only defense against the pathogens in the intestines. The epithelial layer is a physical barrier, whereas various proteases secreted into the lumen act as chemical barriers. Together, they form the first line of defense. The gut microbiota is closely associated with both the intestinal epithelium and GALT and plays a vital role in the development of the gut defense mechanisms.

Biological Plausibility

The role of gut microbiota in immune development is biologically feasible as they colonize the intestines right at birth and co-exist in close vicinity to the immune cells. They provide antigenic stimulation to the early immune cells and play a crucial role in their development.

The defense mechanisms of a newborn's gut differ markedly from adults. The first line of defense is not fully functional as the intestinal epithelium has higher permeability, and the secretion of proteases is not fully developed. The gut immune system encounters very few antigens during the fetal period, due to which it is not adequately trained. The neonatal antigen presenting cells (APCs) have reduced MHC-II expression. Both Th1 and Th2 responses are deficient. Their cytokine production is poor in comparison to adults, particularly for Th-1 response. Studies have shown that IFN-γ production achieves adult levels around the age of five years (Rowe et al., 2000). The function of B lymphocytes also shows differences between adults and infants. Although the number of B cells in the neonate is very high, the maturation to plasma cells is not yet completed, leading to impaired antibody production. The adult-equivalent levels of immunoglobulins are achieved approximately by the age of 10 years (Aksu et al., 2006).

Hygiene Hypothesis

The Hygiene hypothesis links the increased incidence of allergic and autoimmune diseases to the decreased childhood infections in western populations. It was first described by Strachan, who observed an inverse correlation between hay fever and the number of older siblings in more than 17 000 British children born in 1958 (Strachan 1989). In the words of Strachan, written in 1989 –

> These observations do not support suggestions that viral infections, particularly of the respiratory tract, are important precipitants of the expression of atopy. They could, however, be explained if allergic diseases were prevented by infection in early childhood, transmitted by unhygienic contact with older siblings, or acquired prenatally from a mother infected by contact with her older children. Later infection or reinfection by younger siblings might confer additional protection against hay fever. Over the past century declining family sizes, improvements in household amenities, and higher standards of personal cleanliness have reduced the opportunity for cross-infection in young families. This may have resulted in more widespread clinical expression

of atopic disease, emerging earlier in wealthier people, as seems to have occurred for hay fever.

The hygiene hypothesis gained more traction when the off-springs of the first-generation migrants from developing countries with a low incidence of autoimmune disorders such as type-1 diabetes were found to develop these with an incidence similar to the developed host country (Bodansky et al. 1992). This observation extended the hygiene hypothesis from the purview of allergic disorders to autoimmune diseases. The helminth parasites have also been shown to protect against atopy, especially Schistosoma and Necator americanus. The reason behind these observations is that lack of childhood exposure to infectious agents leads to poor development of immune tolerance. The gut microbiota, too, helps in the development of immune tolerance.

Let us know the scientific evidence about how the gut microbiota helps in the transition from the immature gut immune system of a neonate to the robust one of adults and in the development of immune tolerance.

Evidence from Animal Studies

Most of the knowledge regarding the effects of gut microbiota on the immune system comes from studies on germ-free animals. Germ-free mice do not harbor any microorganisms in their intestines or other body surfaces and are helpful in investigating how the intestinal microbiota can shape the developing immune system.

Studies on germ-free animals have shown that the absence of microbial stimulation has profound effects on the development of both the gut innate as well as adaptive immune systems. The villus capillaries of germ-free mice are poorly developed compared to the wild mice suggesting that intestinal bacteria are required for full intestinal blood vessel development (Stappenbeck et al., 2002). Studies have shown that microbes play an essential role in promoting B cell development in Peyer's Patches and drive the production of mucosal IgA antibodies (Shroff, Meslin & Cebra 1995). Germ-free mice produce lesser IgA antibodies than conventional mice and have decreased numbers of circulating B and T lymphocytes (Cebra, 1999).

Several bacterial species and their antigens are required to develop the gut immune system. The gut microbiota also contributes to the development of intraepithelial lymphocytes (IELs), as evidenced by the fact that numbers of IELs are reduced 10-fold in germ-free mice compared to conventional mice

(Mowat, 2003), and the IELs from the germ-free mice lack the cytotoxic activity (Lefrancois and Goodman, 1989).

Gut bacteria play an essential role in the development of immune tolerance. An external antigen in the intestinal lumen can pass through the epithelium via M-cells. M cells are specialized cells in the intestinal epithelium, present in relation to the Peyer's patches. They allow the migration of the antigens (transcytosis) from the intestinal lumen to the lamina propria. The dendritic cells in the lamina propria present these antigens to the naïve T-cells. This leads to the induction of the transcription factor FoxP3 and the differentiation of naïve T cells to the regulatory T cell (T-regs). T-regs produce anti-inflammatory cytokine IL-10, which suppresses the further activation of the immune cascade.

Gut microbiota helps in the development of immune tolerance primarily by increasing the number of T regs. *Lactobacillus reuteri* and *Lactobacillus casei* are shown to increase the production of Tregs (Smits et al. 2005). *Bifidobacterium infantis* has also been shown to increase the Tregs in healthy human volunteers (Konieczna et al. 2012).

The gut microbiota metabolites also play a role in immune tolerance. Acetate, an SCFA, induces Foxp3 expression in naïve T-cells leading to increased maturation to T regs. It has been shown to reduce allergy in mice (Zeng and Chi 2015). Acetate feeding leads to marked suppression of airway disease in a mouse model for human asthma (Thorburn et al. 2015). However, the most important way gut microbiota helps in immune tolerance is probably by providing a large number of antigens to the early immune cells to fine-tune their functions and responses.

Evidence from Human Studies

The increased incidence of allergic disorders and asthma in children born with cesarean section (CS) provided the first indication of the involvement of gut microbiota in these disorders. A number of observational studies have linked cesarean delivery with the increased incidence of asthma (Xu et al. 2001). A recent systematic review analyzing data from 37 studies found that CS increased the risk of childhood asthma with a statistically significant relative risk of 1.2 (Darabi et al. 2019).

The earliest investigations into the role of the gut microbiota in allergic diseases began in the 1990s. They involved healthy one-year-olds in Estonia, where the prevalence of childhood allergy was low, and in Sweden, where allergy prevalence was high. It found that Lactobacilli were more prevalent among Estonian children and *C. difficile* in Swedish children. Following this, the first study comparing the fecal microbiota composition of allergic and healthy children was conducted. It found that allergic children in both countries had reduced lactobacilli and increased facultative aerobic microorganisms, like coliforms in Estonia and *S. aureus* in Sweden (Björkstén et al. 1999). Another study by the same group in 2001 found a lower prevalence of bifidobacteria and enterococci and a higher prevalence of *S. aureus* during the first year of life among children who later developed allergic diseases (Björkstén et al. 2001).

In a recent prospective study, the researchers compared the fecal microbiota of 440 children at various time points from birth until school age. They found that bacterial species during infancy were differentially abundant among children who did or did not develop allergic diseases (AD) at school age. Lachnobacterium and Faecalibacterium were decreased throughout infancy among children who developed AD. And, Lachnospira and Dialister were reduced among children who developed asthma (Galazzo et al. 2020). Similar findings were also observed in the Canadian Healthy Infant Longitudinal Development (CHILD) Study, which revealed Lachnospira and Faecalibacterium to be decreased among children who developed allergic wheeze at the age of 1 year (Subbarao et al. 2015).

Both Lachnospira and Lachnobacterium found to be reduced in children with allergic disorders, produce acetate. Faecalibacterium also has anti-inflammatory effects, which occur through the production of butyrate and a microbial anti-inflammatory molecule. These observations again support the role of gut microbiota in allergic disorders.

Studies in adults have also shown similar findings. Individuals with allergic rhinitis, asthma, and food allergy are shown to have altered gut microbiome compared to healthy individuals.

Clinical Trials

Clinical trials using various probiotic formulations have been conducted for the prevention as well as treatment of allergic disorders. The trials to prevent childhood asthma and allergy have shown mixed results. The initial studies used probiotics in pregnant women during the last weeks of pregnancy to find their effect on the newborns' gut microbiome. The RCT by Ismail et al. found no difference in the diversity of infants' fecal microbiota whose mothers did or did not receive the probiotic Lactobacillus supplementation (Ismail et al. 2012). However, when the probiotics were given both to pregnant mothers and newborns, they increased the microbial diversity and were found to prevent eczema and atopic dermatitis. This beneficial effect of probiotics lasted even up to 2 years of age (Kukkonen et al. 2007). Another RCT investigating the probiotic supplementation to mothers during late pregnancy and lactation without administration to infants did not show benefit in preventing allergic diseases at one year of age (Wickens et al. 2018). Thus, probiotic supplementation given to infants is shown to reduce the incidence of childhood eczema and atopy.

The next set of studies investigated the long-term effects of probiotic supplementation. An RCT published in 2015 found no difference in fecal microbiota composition at six years of age in infants who received probiotics during the first year of life compared to those who did not (Rutten et al. 2015).

Various probiotics have been studied in the treatment of allergic diseases. A combination of Lactobacillus and Bifidobacterium has been shown to reduce the symptoms of allergic rhinitis and improve the quality of life in adults (Denis-Wall et al. 2017). Another RCT of 425 patients using probiotic Lactobacillus in addition to loratadine (an H1 receptor blocker) showed increased benefits (Costa et al. 2014).

Current Practice

Although the RCTs have shown the benefits of probiotics, they are currently not recommended for the prevention or treatment of allergic diseases. At present, they are used mainly in clinical trials.

To conclude, gut microbiota plays an essential role in the early development of the immune system. The gut microbiome of infants who go on to develop allergic diseases lacks certain bacteria such as Lachnobacterium and Faecalibacterium even before the disease onset. Probiotic supplementation during early neonatal life increases microbial diversity and reduces allergic diseases, but the effect lasts only until two years of age. Probiotics also showed symptomatic improvement in adults with allergic rhinitis but the current guidelines do not recommend them for routine use.

Chapter 4

Gut Microbiota: Role in Metabolic Diseases

Goals

1. Understanding the terms dysbiosis, endotoxemia, and low-grade inflammation
2. To know about the role of gut microbiota in chronic inflammation and lifestyle diseases
3. To know about the role of gut microbiota in satiety signaling
4. To know the current clinical applications

Ischemic heart disease and stroke are the most common cause of death worldwide (WHO Global Health Estimates 2000-2019). The metabolic disorders, including obesity, diabetes, and metabolic syndrome, are precursors to ischemic cardiac and cerebrovascular diseases. These disorders are also known as lifestyle diseases because the rise in their incidence is correlated with the change in diet and lifestyle habits over the last few decades.

The link between the gut microbiota and metabolic disorders is the most significant role the gut microbiome plays in human health and diseases. The fact that lifestyle factors such as diet and exercise profoundly impact the composition and function of the gut microbiome further highlights this connection. Let us know how the alterations in the gut microbiota are associated with metabolic diseases and the scientific evidence behind them.

Biological Plausibility

Endotoxemia and Low-Grade Inflammation

The intestinal epithelium forms an effective barrier to the passage of substances from the intestinal lumen to the lymphatic or vascular system. As learned in chapter 2, this barrier is not a fixed entity, and the intestinal permeability can change in response to various stimuli.

The cell walls of Gram-negative bacteria are made up of lipopolysaccharide (LPS). Most bacteria belonging to the phylum proteobacteria have LPS. When these bacteria die, the LPS is released in the intestinal lumen and absorbed in the circulation. The increased intestinal permeability allows a larger amount of LPS to enter the bloodstream leading to increased plasma LPS levels, termed *endotoxemia*. Endotoxemia is a function of two factors: increased availability of LPS due to alteration in the gut microbiota and increased intestinal permeability. The alteration in the gut microbiota composition associated with a disease is known as *dysbiosis*.

The LPS, once absorbed, is recognized by the toll-like receptor (TLR) -4 present on the cell membrane of macrophages and dendritic cells. The interaction between LPS and TLR-4 activates the downstream signal pathways, ultimately leading to the activation of nuclear factor-κB (NF-κB). The NF-κB is a transcription factor that upregulates the genes responsible for the production and secretion of inflammatory markers such as cytokines, chemokines, and cell adhesion molecules. Thus, the increased absorption of the LPS, either due to increased availability or increased intestinal permeability, leads to increased inflammatory markers in the systemic circulation. This phenomenon is termed low-grade systemic inflammation. It must be noted that the inflammation in this setting is much weaker (around 15 times) than that occurs in sepsis, and hence it is termed as low-grade.

Inflammation is a normal process of the host defense system. However, an unresolved (chronic) low-grade inflammatory response due to endotoxemia leads to a state of persistent systemic inflammation that is the precursor to lifestyle diseases, including type 2 diabetes mellitus (T2DM), non-alcoholic fatty liver disease (NAFLD), and obesity.

We understood that dysbiosis and increased intestinal permeability lead to endotoxemia which causes a state of low-grade inflammation. Dysbiosis has a double impact because it increases both intestinal permeability and LPS production (Figure 4.1).

Insulin Resistance

Insulin resistance is the underlying pathophysiology of metabolic disorders, including diabetes. Diabetes is characterized by increased blood glucose levels and its after-effects. The blood glucose level is tightly regulated. Hormones such as insulin and incretins decrease blood glucose, whereas glucagon and corticosteroids increase it. Diabetes can be caused by multiple mechanisms involving abnormal secretion or function of any of these hormones. However, the most common of them, type 2 diabetes, occurs due to the reduced ability of insulin to act on its target tissues. This inability is termed insulin resistance.

Insulin is a pleiotropic hormone. It has diverse functions, which include facilitating nutrient transportation into cells, regulation of gene expression, and modification of enzymatic activity. These functions are carried out in various organs, the most important of which are skeletal muscle, liver, and adipose tissue. In skeletal muscle, insulin promotes glucose uptake by stimulating translocation of the GLUT 4 glucose transporter to the plasma membrane, leading to a reduction in blood glucose levels. In the liver, insulin inhibits gluconeogenesis and, therefore, leads to decreased hepatic glucose production. Gluconeogenesis is the process of the conversion of amino acids into glucose. In adipose tissue, insulin results in decreased hormone-sensitive lipase activity and reduces the breakdown of triglycerides into free fatty acids. This anti-lipolytic effect inhibits free fatty acid efflux from adipocytes and reduces circulating free fatty acids. When insulin resistance sets in, these functions are impaired, leading to decreased glucose uptake in skeletal muscles and increased production from the liver, and ultimately increased blood glucose levels.

Insulin acts via a set of receptors termed insulin receptor substrate (IRS). These are a family of 4 different receptors, IRS1-4. IRS are transmembrane tyrosine kinase receptors. Tyrosine kinase receptors are activated when the ligand binds them, leading to the autophosphorylation of particular tyrosine residues. This initiates the downstream pathways, which ultimately carry out the various functions. When insulin binds to the IRS, it leads to tyrosine phosphorylation of IRS, thereby initiating signal transduction. When instead of tyrosine, IRS-1 is alternatively phosphorylated at serine 307, the downstream signaling is inhibited, and insulin resistance occurs.

The Link between Inflammation and Insulin Resistance

The persistent low-grade inflammation leads to the phosphorylation of IRS-1 at serine 307 and, thus, to insulin resistance. The pro-inflammatory markers lead to the activation of enzymes known as serine kinases. Serine kinases phosphorylate a protein at the particular serine residue. In the case of IRS-1, they phosphorylate at serine 307. Serine kinases that phosphorylate IRS-1 include I kappa B kinase beta (Ikkb) in the NFκB pathway and C-Jun N-terminal kinase 1 (Jnk1) in the JNK/AP-1 pathway.

To summarize, alteration in gut microbiota (dysbiosis) leads to endotoxemia. The LPS-TLR4 interaction activates inflammatory pathways, ultimately leading to phosphorylation of IRS-1 at serine 307. It inhibits the downstream signaling of IRS and blocks the action of insulin on target organs, causing insulin resistance (Figure 4.1).

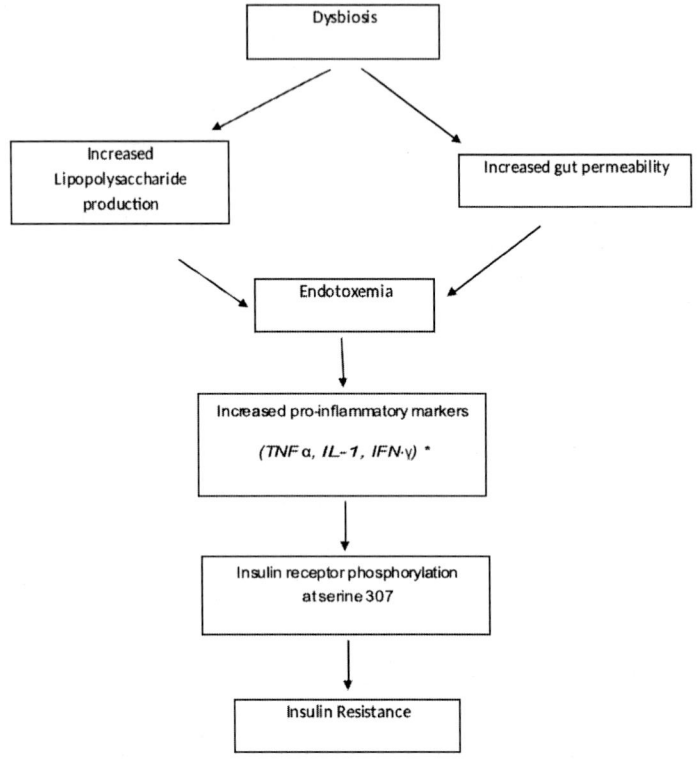

* $TNF\alpha$, Tumor necrosis factor-α; IL-1, interleukin-1; IFN-γ, Interferon- γ

Figure 4.1. Pathophysiological basis of how dysbiosis results in insulitn resistance.

Dysbiosis

Dysbiosis is the alteration of gut microbiota in relation to a disease. A normal or healthy gut microbiome has few salient features. It is characterized by an abundance of bacteria that can ferment complex carbohydrates, low numbers of proteobacteria, and abundant bifidobacteria. But, the most important feature of the healthy gut microbiome is 'diversity.' The reduced microbial diversity is usually the first sign of gut dysbiosis and is a feature of almost all the diseases associated with an alteration in gut microbiota.

One of the most common parameters used to indicate species diversity in an ecosystem is *Simpson's Diversity Index*. Its value varies from 0, which means no diversity, to 1, which means infinite diversity. Although originally devised for ecological studies, Simpson's index is widely used to indicate gut microbiota diversity. The formula to calculate it is beyond the scope of this book. Let us remember that Simpson's Index is a common method to indicate the diversity of gut microbiota.

The other terminologies which are commonly used in studies are *alpha-diversity* and *beta-diversity*. Let us understand them with an example. Suppose there are two lakes, Lake 1 and Lake 2. Lake 1 has ten different fish species, and Lake 2 has 100. When we talk about each lake individually, we are talking about alpha-diversity. For example, for the purpose of understanding, we can say the alpha-diversity of Lake 1 is ten and Lake 2 is 100, which means the fauna of Lake 2 is more diverse. But when we compare the different fish species found in the two lakes, then it is termed beta-diversity. In the current example, if all the ten species found in Lake 1 are different from the 100 species found in Lake 2, then it means that the beta diversity between them is high.

In the context of the gut microbiome, when an individual's gut microbiota is described as diverse or less diverse, it is alpha-diversity. And when the gut-flora of two individuals or different populations is compared with each other, it is beta-diversity. If the Indian gut microbiome differs markedly from an American, there is high beta-diversity between the two. At the same time, any one of them may have high alpha-diversity depending upon the number of different bacterial species they harbor. It is paramount to note that it is the alpha-diversity that matters from an individual's point of view. When a study shows that the gut microbiome of diabetics is less diverse than non-diabetics, it is talking about the alpha-diversity.

Gut Microbiota and Satiety Signaling

Satiety is the sensation of fullness and satisfaction one feels on eating food. An impaired satiety signaling can lead to overconsumption of calories and obesity. The gut microbiota plays a pivotal role in the satiety signaling in our body.

Peptide YY

Peptide YY is a hormone secreted by the enteroendocrine L-cells in the ileum. It is secreted in response to the presence of fats and amino acids in the small intestine. Peptide YY reaches the brain and delivers the feeling of satiety. Its receptors (Y1 and Y2) are located in the area prostrema, the nucleus of the solitary tract, and the dorsal motor nucleus of the vagus in the central nervous system (CNS). It also slows gastric emptying and reduces gastric acid and pancreatic enzyme secretions. So, when we consume food, fats and amino acids reach the small intestine leading to the release of Peptide YY, which tells us to stop through its actions on GIT and CNS.

How does the gut microbiota play a role in satiety? The L-cells that secrete the Peptide YY have G-protein coupled receptors. Butyrate activates these receptors leading to the secretion of Peptide YY. We know that butyrate is a gut microbiota metabolite exclusively produced by the action of microbial enzymes on complex carbohydrates. Thus, butyrate production, which leads to Peptide YY secretion, is another mechanism by which gut microbiota prevents obesity and metabolic diseases.

Secondary Bile Acids

Bile acids are secreted by the liver. They reach the duodenum via the bile duct and help absorb dietary fats. The bile acids secreted by the liver are known as primary bile acids. Cholic acid (CA) and Chenodeoxycholic acid (CDCA) are primary bile acids. The primary bile acids are converted by the gut microbiota to the secondary bile acids in the ileum and colon. The microbial hydrolases act on the CA and CDCA and convert them to Deoxycholic acid and lithocholic acid.

(Bacterial hydrolases)

Cholic Acid ⟶ Deoxycholic Acid

Chenodeoxycholic Acid ⟶ Lithocholic acid

The bile acids helphuman metabolism in 3 ways:

1. Bile acids act on the L-cell in the ileum through a receptor TGR-5, a G-protein coupled receptor that leads to the secretion of GLP-1. TGR-5 has the most binding affinity to Lithocholic acid. GLP-1 is an incretin hormone that leads to insulin secretion from the pancreas and slows gastric emptying. Both these factors help lower blood glucose levels (Xie et al. 2021).
2. Bile acids act on a receptor present on the intestinal epithelial cells, known as the FXR receptor, and activate it. FXR is a nuclear factor. On activation, it moves to the nucleus and regulates gene expression. Bile acids are the natural ligands of the FXR in the human body. FXR has a wide range of functions, including a role in liver regeneration. As far as metabolic functions are concerned, it primarily influences lipid and glucose balance. FXR activation leads to decreased hepatic triglyceride synthesis, reduces gluconeogenesis, and increases insulin sensitivity (Wang et al. 2008, Jiao et al. 2015).
3. Recently, bile acids have been found to directly induce satiety. They are shown to be present in the CNS. In an experimental study, bile acids injected arterially into the mice led to anorexia (Perino et al. 2021). This central action of bile acids is also mediated through TGR-5 present in the areas of the brain controlling satiety.

Evidence from Animal Studies

Animal studies have shown that a high-fat diet can cause endotoxemia. Cani et al. observed that serum levels of LPS in mice after a 4-week high-fat diet were similar to that of mice continuously infused with LPS for four weeks. They termed this high-fat diet induced increase in serum LPS as metabolic endotoxemia (Cani et al. 2007). The metabolic endotoxemia can lead to persistent low-grade inflammation, ultimately leading to the development of insulin resistance and metabolic disorders.

Another landmark study in 2006 proved the role of gut microbiota in the development of obesity. In this study, the cecal microbiota of the obese and the lean mice were transplanted each to a group of germ-free mice. Both the recipient groups received a similar diet, and there was no difference in the amount of diet consumed by the two groups. After 14 days, the total body fat was higher in germ-free mice transplanted with the obese gut microbiota (Turnbaugh et al. 2006). This study showed that obesity can be transmitted from one organism to another like an infectious disease.

Evidence from Human Studies

Gut microbiota has been shown to be altered in individuals with T2DM and obesity. The reduction in gut microbial diversity is the most common and consistent finding. Two large metagenome-wide association studies reported that subjects with type 2 diabetes mellitus had gut dysbiosis, a lower proportion of butyrate-producing *Clostridiales* (*Roseburia* and *Faecalibacterium prausnitzii*), and a greater proportion of *Clostridiales* that do not produce butyrate. Clostridiales is a class of bacteria in the phylum Firmicutes. This finding suggests a protective role of butyrate-producing bacteria against T2DM (Karlson et al. 2013, Qin et al. 2010). Gut microbiota alteration even predates the occurrence of diabetes. In a large population-based Swedish study including more than 1500 subjects, gut microbiota was found to be altered in individuals with pre-diabetes. The reduction in butyrate production was again the most critical finding (Wu et al. 2020).

In obesity, apart from reduced microbial diversity, an increased number of Firmicutes and decreased number of Bacteroidetes have been found leading to increased Firmicutes/ Bacteroidetes ratio. An increase in Firmicutes probably leads to increased energy absorption from the food. However, one of the Firmicutes, *Faecalibacterium prausnitzii,* is reduced in obese individuals (Mörkl et al. 2018). Thus, Firmicutes as a whole may increase in obesity but the individual species behave differently. Various studies have stressed on the role of the Firmicutes/Bacteroidetes (F/B) ratio as a marker of obesity and the quality of the gut microbiome. However, contradictory findings such as increased Bacteroidetes in individuals with T2DM and increased abundance of Firmicutes on a high-fiber diet which is associated with weight reduction, have cast doubt on this generalization. I refrain from giving importance to the F/B ratio and advise you to be cautious about it.

Bifidobacterium is reduced in obese individuals. Breast-fed infants have been found to develop fewer lifestyle diseases. The secret ingredient in the mother's milk that makes it possible is Bifidobacterium. A study by kalliomaki et al. determined whether early gut microbiota composition can impact future weight gain during early childhood. They selected 25 overweight and 24 normal-weight children at seven years of age who were enrolled in a different prospective study as infants. These children had fecal samples stored during infancy. The gut microbial analysis of the stored fecal samples found that Bifidobacterium numbers during infancy were higher in children who were normal-weight at seven years. At the same time, the stored fecal samples of obese children had increased *Staphylococcus aureus* (Kalliomaki et al. 2008). Thus, the presence of Bifidobacterium in gut microbiota during infancy can be protective against childhood obesity.

Clinical Trials

The next question is whether alteration in gut microbiota has been shown to directly lead to or cure metabolic disorders in humans.

In an interesting serendipitous observation, a patient with recurrent *C. difficile* infection received fecal microbiota transplantation (FMT) from an overweight donor. He recovered but had an unintentional weight gain of 34 pounds despite a medically supervised diet and exercise program. The weight gain was attributed to the change in gut microbiota due to FMT, which cured the infection but also altered the patient's metabolism. However, the gut microbiome analysis was not performed to document the changes associated with obesity (Alang & Kelly 2015).

In another study, fecal bacteria from lean and healthy people were transplanted to individuals with metabolic syndrome. Six weeks after the microbiota transplant, insulin sensitivity improved and butyrate-producing bacteria increased in the recipients' gut microbiota (Vireze et al. 2012). In a similar study, Dutch scientists performed FMT from a lean donor to obese men with metabolic syndrome, which increased the insulin sensitivity of the recipients. The gut microbial diversity also increased, suggesting that the fecal transplant altered the metabolism through the changes in the gut microbiome. The benefits lasted till 18 weeks after the procedure (Koott et al. 2017).

In an RCT, 24 obese men and women with insulin resistance were recruited. Half of them received specially prepared frozen capsules containing stool from the four lean donors and the other half received a placebo. After 12 weeks, the study found that the fecal microbiota treatment using capsules was safe and tolerable, and the subjects had acquired gut bacteria that resembled the donors' (Yu et al. 2020). But overall, there was no improvement in metabolic health as compared to the control group.

Probiotics

Probiotics are live organisms that provide health benefits when consumed in adequate amounts. Multiple studies have explored their role in metabolic disorders.

A proof-of-concept study in 2015 evaluated the effect of four-week daily supplementation with Lactobacillus reuteri on insulin secretion in healthy volunteers. The researchers found increased GLP-1, and insulin secretion in response to glucose in these subjects. But it did not alter peripheral and hepatic insulin sensitivity, body weight, and circulating inflammatory cytokines in the recipients (Simon et al. 2015).

A meta-analysis of RCTs conducted before 2016 found that probiotics lead to minor improvements in various metabolic parameters. In overweight patients, probiotics led to improvements in weight, BMI, waist circumference, and body fat mass. In T2 DM, they improved fasting glucose, HBA1C, and insulin resistance. However, the studies included were heterogenous, the improvements were minor, and patients also received adjunctive treatments or lifestyle modifications (Koutnikova et al. 2019).

A recent RCT studying the impact of 24-week synbiotic supplementation found no improvement in inflammatory markers and glycemic control in patients with type-2 diabetes. Synbiotics are a combination of probiotics and prebiotics (Kanazawa et al. 2021). Another placebo-controlled trial of a multi-specie probiotic given for six months to patients with both diabetes and obesity showed no benefits in blood glucose levels (Horvath et al. 2020). An RCT conducted on obese pregnant women without diabetes showed a reduction in fasting blood glucose levels in the probiotic group, but there was no difference in the incidence of gestational diabetes between the two groups (Asgharian et al. 2020). However, a recent RCT showed the benefits of probiotic *Saccharomyces boulardii* in individuals with obesity. A 60-day supplementation in 12 obese individuals led to a significant reduction in weight and body fat, while the placebo arm didn't have any effect (Rondanelli et al. 2021).

To summarize, probiotics have shown clinically insignificant benefits in diabetes and obesity. An occasional study has shown the benefit, but more scientific evidence is needed before they can be routinely prescribed for metabolic disorders.

Current Practice

Clinical guidelines do not recommend gut microbiota therapy in individuals with obesity or diabetes.

Both probiotics and FMT are used only in clinical trials currently.

To conclude, alteration in gut microbiota leads to metabolic disorders as dysbiosis results in endotoxemia, ultimately leading to insulin resistance. Transfer of gut microbiota from obese subjects is shown to increase the recipient's body weight and fat mass in both animals and human studies. Probiotics and FMT have shown improvement in insulin sensitivity, but no consistent clinically meaningful benefits are shown as yet.

Chapter 5

Gut Microbiota: Role in Cardiovascular Disease

Goals

1. To know about the pathophysiology of atherosclerosis
2. Understanding the role of TMAO in atherosclerosis and cardiovascular diseases
3. Understanding the role of gut microbiota in TMAO production
4. To know the current clinical applications

Cardiovascular diseases (CVDs) are the leading causes of death globally. According to a WHO report, an estimated 17.9 million people died from CVDs in 2019. CVDs accounted for 32% of all deaths, 85% of which occurred due to heart attack and stroke.

Biological Plausibility

The underlying pathophysiology of CVDs is the development of atherosclerosis. Atherosclerosis is the thickening or hardening of the arteries. It is characterized by the formation of plaques in the arterial wall. The atherosclerotic plaques are formed in the innermost layer of the arterial wall known as intima. Over time, the plaque leads to the narrowing and, ultimately, occlusion of the arterial lumen leading to myocardial infarction and stroke.

The initial step of atherosclerosis development is foam cell formation. Foam cell is the macrophage present in the arterial intima that is laden with lipids. The atherogenic process starts with the migration of circulating monocytes from the blood into the arterial intima, where they differentiate into macrophages. Low-Density Lipoprotein (LDL) enters the arterial wall through a receptor called Scavenger receptor class B type 1 (SR-B1) (Huang et al. 2019). The binding of LDL-1 to SR-B1 leads to the internalization of LDL into the endothelial cells and then migration into the intima by transcytosis.

The mice with the SR-B1 gene knocked out show reduced LDL accumulation in the intima. The LDL accumulated into the intima is oxidized by various enzymes such as myeloperoxidase and Lipoxygenase etc., to form oxidized LDL (Cyrus et al. 1999).

The macrophages, already present in the arterial intima, bind the oxidized LDL through a receptor present on their cell membranes - CD36. The CD-36 is a scavenger receptor that helps absorb long-chain fatty acids. The CD-36-bound oxidized LDL enters the macrophages. The internalized oxidized LDL increases the expression of CD36 on the macrophage cell membrane, which leads to more oxidized LDL uptake. This feed-forward signal by the oxidized LDL is also called as 'eat me signal.' The macrophages also secrete oxidants, including myeloperoxidase, which oxidizes the LDL present in the intima and thus, enlarges the pool of available oxidized LDL. LDL (non-oxidized) can also enter the macrophages in the intima, but that process is very slow, and thus oxidation of LDL is a key step in atherosclerosis. The interaction between CD36 and oxidized LDL also causes the secretion of cytokines that recruit immune cells in the arterial intima and lead to the inflammation of the arterial wall, which further narrows the arterial lumen leading to CVDs.

TMAO is a gut microbiota metabolite. It is produced by the action of microbial enzymes on dietary choline, lecithin, and L-carnitine. TMAO is shown to be associated with atherosclerosis and CVD. Increased TMAO levels correlate with an increased risk of myocardial infarction and stroke. Prospective cohort studies have shown that increased plasma TMAO levels predicted an elevated risk of myocardial infarction, stroke, and death in patients with pre-existing atherosclerosis. A 3-year follow-up of 4,007 patients undergoing elective coronary angiography revealed a significant association between elevated plasma TMAO levels and increased risk of stroke, myocardial infarction, or death (Tang et al. 2013).

How does TMAO lead to increased atherosclerosis and CVD? There are various proposed mechanisms by which TMAO promotes atherosclerosis (Yang et al. 2019).

1. TMAO increases the expression of CD-36 on macrophages, leading to increased uptake of oxidized LDL and formation of foam cells.
2. TMAO is associated with increased pro-inflammatory markers and platelet activity, leading to an increased risk of thrombosis.
3. TMAO reduces the bile acid synthesis in the liver. As cholesterol is the prime substrate for bile acid synthesis, it leads to decreased cholesterol utilization in the liver. More cholesterol is then secreted

in the lipoprotein particles from the liver, leading to increased atherosclerosis.

Evidence from Animal Studies

Animal experiments have primarily looked into the mechanisms by which the TMAO accelerates the development of atherosclerosis.

In one study, mice were fed a high-fat diet with or without TMAO for eight weeks. Atherosclerosis progression was higher in TMAO-fed mice. TMAO also enhanced CD36 expression and pro-inflammatory cytokines in atherosclerotic plaques. In the second stage of the experiment, MAP kinase and Janus kinase inhibitors were given to the mice. Both these inhibitors decreased the TMAO-induced CD-36 expression. The study concluded that the effect of TMAO on CD-36 expression is mediated via MAP kinase and Janus kinase pathways (Geng et al. 2018).

TMAO levels are shown to be associated with higher levels of inflammatory markers. Obese mice have higher plasma TMAO levels as well as increased pro-inflammatory cytokines, including TNF-α, and IL-1β, while decreased expression of the anti-inflammatory cytokine IL-10. TMAO-mediated inflammation occurs by the activation of the inflammasome pathway (Chen et al. 2017).

The effect of TMAO on thrombosis was demonstrated in an elegant mice study. TMAO was infused intraperitoneally in the test mice. It led to increased plasma levels of TMAO and thrombosis of the internal carotid artery at the site of an experimentally induced injury. The increased platelet activity in the presence of TMAO occurred due to a several-fold increase in the release of intracellular calcium. TMAO augments the rise in platelet intracellular calcium levels in response to the vessel wall injury, leading to increased platelet aggregation and thrombus formation (Zhu et al. 2016).

TMAO also inhibits bile acid synthesis. In a Chinese study, mice were fed a regular or TMAO-containing diet for eight weeks. The TMAO-fed mice showed increased development of aortic atherosclerosis. The bile acid synthesis was reduced in the TMAO-fed mice. Mice liver tissue was analyzed to find the reason for reduced bile acid synthesis. The expression of Cyp7a1, which catalyzes the first rate-limiting step of bile acid synthesis from cholesterol, was reduced in the TMAO-fed mice (Ding et al. 2018).

All these studies demonstrate how the TMAO promotes atherosclerosis and CVDs. The role of gut microbiota in the production of TMAO has also been established in the studies conducted on germ-free mice. Germ-free mice fed with choline could not produce TMAO. These mice were then co-habited with the wild-type mice harboring gut microbiota. This led to the development of gut microbiota in germ-free mice. Now, they were again fed the choline-containing diet, which, on this occasion, led to the TMAO production. Thus, the germ-free mice that did not produce TMAO earlier produced it when they harbored gut microbiota (Wang et al. 2011). This finding proves that the gut microbiota is necessary for the production of TMAO.

Evidence from Human Studies

Many human studies have conclusively shown TMAO to be associated with CVD and established the role of gut microbiota in TMAO production.

A landmark study published in Nature showed that the gut microbiota metabolism of dietary lipid, phosphatidylcholine, promotes cardiovascular diseases. In this study, a metabolomic profile of plasma was done in healthy adults to identify metabolites that could predict CVD development over the next three years. A metabolomics study strives to find all the metabolites in the given biological sample, which in this study was plasma. The three metabolites which could predict CVD were TMAO, betaine, and choline (Wang et al. 2011). All of them are produced by the metabolism of phosphatidylcholine in the human body. Phosphatidylcholine is present in both plants as well as animal-based foods. However, as much as 65% of it is obtained from eggs, meat, and fish in a study conducted on Norwegian CVD patients (Van Parys et al. 2021). Initially, phosphatidylcholine is metabolized to choline and betaine in the intestines. The gut microbial enzymes then catabolize them to form the gas TMA, which is rapidly absorbed and reaches the liver. In the liver, TMA is metabolized by the hepatic enzyme flavin monooxygenase-3 (FMO3) to form TMAO. Wang et al. also measured the levels of choline, betaine, and TMAO in a separate cohort of 1876 patients to validate their findings. Elevated levels of all of them were found to be associated with CVD in a dose-dependent manner.

Another study found that increased plasma TMAO was associated with an increased risk of a major adverse cardiovascular event (hazard ratio for highest vs. lowest TMAO quartile, 2.54) even after adjustment for traditional risk factors (Tang et al. 2013). Since then, many studies have shown an association between TMAO and CVDs. Similar findings were observed in a recent meta-analysis of 19 prospective studies (Heianza et al. 2017). Individuals with elevated plasma TMAO (relative risk 1.62) and TMAO precursors had a higher risk of CVDs.

The role of gut microbiota in human TMAO metabolism was shown in a landmark study. In this study, healthy subjects were given a phosphatidylcholine challenge followed by measurement of TMAO, betaine, and choline, all of which were elevated. The subjects were then given antibiotics ciprofloxacin and metronidazole for one week, following which the phosphatidylcholine challenge was repeated. Plasma levels of TMAO were markedly suppressed during the second challenge. A third challenge was performed after one month of the antibiotic withdrawal, which again showed elevated TMAO levels. These findings corroborated the observations in the mice and proved that gut microbiota is essential for the production of TMAO in humans as well (Tang et al. 2013).

Trials on Reducing TMAO

TMAO reduction is a promising strategy to prevent and treat CVDs considering its role in atherosclerosis progression and association with important clinical outcomes such as myocardial infarction, stroke, and death.

The TMAO production can be inhibited by altering the gut microbiota using antibiotics, as shown in the study by Tang et al. Still, long-term antibiotic treatment can result in various adverse events, including intestinal dysbiosis. Therefore, antibiotics are not a feasible strategy to reduce TMAO production in clinical practice. The use of long-term probiotics to achieve a healthier gut microbiota and reduction in TMAO levels is a safer and more viable option. In a study of 90 individuals with CVD risk factors a probiotic product, Lacto-fermented Annurca apple puree, was found to reduce plasma TMAO and raise HDL cholesterol levels (Tenore et al. 2019). However, a study with the multi-strain probiotic VSL#3 in non-obese males on a high-fat diet did not reduce the TMAO. In this RCT, healthy adults were divided into two groups and were given a high-fat diet for four weeks. One group received VSL#3 and the other placebo along with the high-fat diet. The increase in TMAO levels after 4 weeks was found to be similar in both groups (Boutagy et al. 2015).

A recent systematic review including 34 studies found that probiotic use was associated with both systolic and diastolic blood pressure reduction and lesser LDL cholesterol levels. However, TMAO levels were not assessed in this systematic review (Dixon et al. 2020). Another RCT published in 2021 did not show any difference in TMAO levels after the phosphatidylcholine challenge between healthy adults who received the probiotics (for four weeks) or placebo. In general, probiotics have not been shown to effectively lower TMAO levels in human studies.

The other strategies to reduce TMAO production include inhibiting FMO3 which converts TMA to TMAO. In mice experiments, it led to abnormally high levels of TMA, which would be harmful to humans. Besides, FMO_3 has other physiological functions in the human body, and thus, inhibiting it is not a helpful strategy.

To summarize, human studies have shown a conclusive association between TMAO and CVDs and the role of gut microbiota in TMAO production. Still, we have not found an effective and safe way to reduce plasma TMAO levels in long term.

Current Practice

The current guidelines do not recommend gut microbiota therapy in preventing or treating cardiovascular diseases either as a stand-alone therapy or as an adjunct to the routinely prescribed treatment.

Probiotics can be used in clinical trials.

The role of FMT should be explored in CVDs.

Chapter 6

Role in Stress and Related Disorders

Goals

1. To know about stress and its impact on gut microbiota
2. To learn about the gut-brain axis
3. To learn about serotonin and its relation to the gut microbiome
4. To know the current clinical applications

What Is Stress ?

Stress biologically is a stimulus that leads to the increased secretion of corticosteroid and sympathomimetic hormones. To learn about the biology of stress, let us go back to our ancestors. The genus Homo originated around 2 million years ago, and the human species Homo sapiens originated 200 000 years back. From then till the advent of agriculture which occurred only about 12000 years ago, humans were primarily hunter-gatherers. Let us imagine a day in the life of one of our hunter-gatherer ancestors. She woke up in the morning and began searching for food. While roaming in the forest, she encountered a wild animal. Her brain rightly perceived it as a danger and directed her adrenals to secrete epinephrine, which leads to sympathetic activation and increases blood circulation, alertness, and muscle activity.
    Armed with these beneficial responses, she ran to safety and saved herself. She might not face any other stressors that day. Now compare it with our modern lives. The danger encountered by our ancestors was real but short-lived. At the same time, we experience continuous or *chronic stress* in our daily lives. Although we have made tremendous scientific and industrial progress over the last few centuries, we are the same as our ancestors at the physiological and psychological levels. Our brain and body respond to stress in a similar fashion. Thus, the continuous or chronic stress we encounter results in persistent activation of our sympathetic system and increased cortisol secretion. This causes elevation of both the blood pressure and blood glucose, leading to lifestyle diseases. While sympathetic system activation increases cardiac contractility and vascular tone, causing elevation of both the

systolic and diastolic blood pressure, the increased cortisol leads to gluconeogenesis and causes muscle protein breakdown to produce more glucose. Thus, chronic stress is as detrimental to human health as chronic inflammation.

Biological Plausibility

Gut-Brain Axis

The human brain and GIT have constant bidirectional cross-talk (Figure 6.1). Each of us has felt irritable and angry when hungry and butterflies in our stomachs when nervous, thereby having a first-hand experience of this interaction.

There are three ways by which this interaction occurs:

1. *Neural pathway*: The Vagus nerve originates in the hindbrain, and its neurons innervate almost the entire digestive system. They form synaptic connections with the neurons of the enteral nervous system (ENS). ENS is the collection of neurons present in the wall of our digestive system. Thus, the signals from our brain relay through the vagus nerve to the ENS and control the gut motility and gut hormone secretion. For example, the butterflies we experience are the perceived intestinal contractions due to the increased gut motility.
2. *Immune pathway*: As already mentioned, GIT is the largest immune organ in the human body. The immune cells in GIT secrete various molecules, called cytokines and prostaglandin E2, which reach the brain via the bloodstream and affect its function.
3. *Endocrine pathway*: Our intestines have more than 20 types of endocrine cells that make them the largest endocrine organ in the human body. The endocrine cells secrete a large variety of hormones which can reach the central nervous system and alter its function. One such example already discussed is the effect of Peptide YY on the satiety signals.

The gut microbiota has an impact on all three pathways. They reside close to the ENS nerve endings and stimulate them directly or via metabolites. Lactobacillus reuteri has been shown to directly modulate sensory nerve endings and alter gut motility and pain perception (Kunze et al. 2009).

Microbiota also produces substances such as GABA and serotonin, which are neurotransmitters and act on both the CNS and ENS. The hydrogen sulfide produced by the microbiota interacts with the vanilloid receptor on nerve endings and modulates gut motility (Schicho et al. 2006). And lastly, the gut microbiota metabolites, SCFAs, also stimulate the sympathetic nervous system (Kimura et al. 2011).

As far as the immune and endocrine pathways are concerned, we have already discussed the role of gut bacteria and GMMs in immune development and enteroendocrine cell stimulation in previous chapters. The role of gut microbiota is so well established in gut-brain interaction that the gut-brain axis is now frequently termed the microbiome-gut-brain axis.

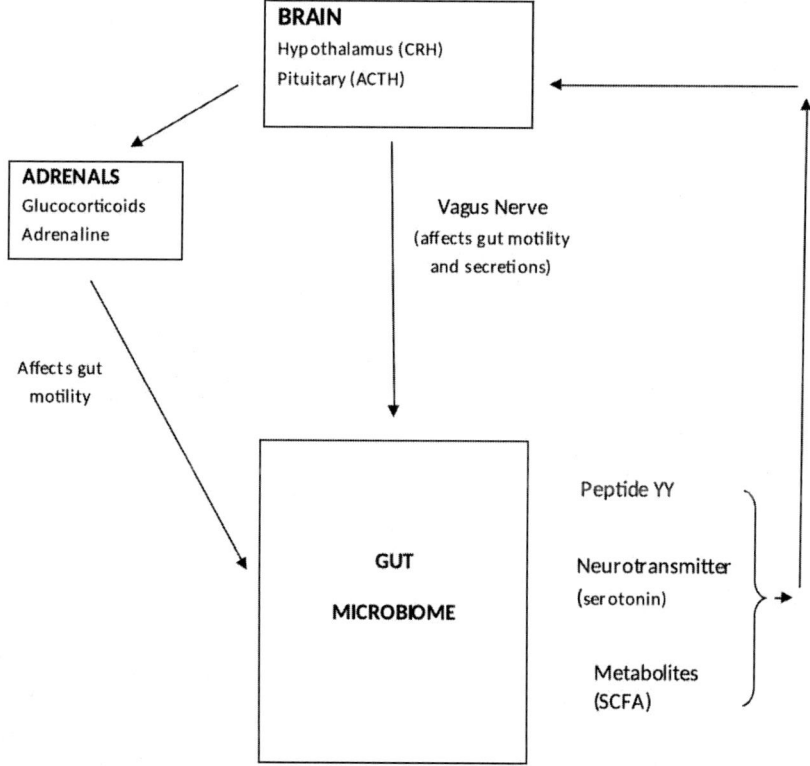

Figure 6.1. Schematic diagram of bi-directional microbiome-gut-brain axis.

Serotonin

Serotonin (5-hydroxy tryptamine or 5-HT) is known as the 'Happy hormone.' It is a neurotransmitter. The elevated serotonin activity in the brain gives the feeling of happiness. The antidepressant drugs, selective serotonin reuptake inhibitors (SSRIs), act by blocking the reuptake of serotonin at the synaptic junctions. This leads to the increased levels and availability of serotonin in the synaptic cleft, which ultimately leads to the antidepressant effect.

More than 90 % of the serotonin in the human body is produced in the gut by the enterochromaffin cells (ECs), and the microbiota plays an important role in this process. Serotonin is produced from tryptophan, an essential amino acid, which must be supplied in the diet. Tryptophan hydroxylase is the key rate-limiting enzyme in the serotonin production pathway.

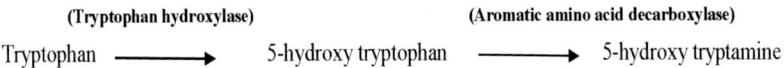

Tryptophan $\xrightarrow{\text{(Tryptophan hydroxylase)}}$ 5-hydroxy tryptophan $\xrightarrow{\text{(Aromatic amino acid decarboxylase)}}$ 5-hydroxy tryptamine

Studies have shown that serum concentrations of 5-HT are substantially reduced in germ-free mice compared to wild mice (Sjögren et al. 2012). In a study published in the journal Cell, Yano et al. showed that spore-forming bacteria leads to increased 5-HT synthesis in the colonic ECs. They performed metabolomics to identify the metabolites that stimulate ECs to produce more serotonin. They identified a set of metabolites, including α-tocopherol, butyrate, *cholate*, *deoxycholate*, propionate, and *tyramine* which stimulated ECs and elevated 5-HT levels (Yano et al. 2015).

Effect of Stress on Gut Microbiota

Stress has a profound impact on gut microbiota. Its effect on the gut microbiome even outlasts the stressful period. This is particularly true of 'early-life stress.' Early-life stress is a severe form of stress which occurs because of situations encountered during childhood. It is also called adverse childhood experiences or "ACEs." These include abuse, neglect, and a non-conducive home environment during childhood or teenage years. It increases the risk of many illnesses, including depression and heart diseases, even after the person has overcome the stressful environment.

Various mice studies have conclusively shown the effect of early stress on the gut microbiota. In one such study, mice were separated from their mothers daily for 3 hours soon after birth to mimic an early-life stress situation. The mice separated from their mothers had an altered gut microbiota compared to the non-separated mice, particularly with reduced bacterial diversity. Besides, the isolated mice had increased stress hormones and pro-inflammatory substances (O'Mahony et al. 2009). In another mice study, scientists found that gut microbiota changes which occur in response to stress are similar to those that occur due to a high-fat diet (Bridgewater et al. 2017).

Human studies comparing the gut microbiome of the individuals who experienced early-life stress to those who didn't have shown similar findings. In a study conducted on healthy pregnant women, half of whom had experienced childhood stressors, researchers found that the women with early-life stress had different gut microbiota than women without such experiences. These women were both physically and psychologically healthy at the time of the study, but still, the early-life stress they experienced had an impact on the gut microbiota even years later. Specifically, they had an increased abundance of the bacterium *Prevotella, which* has been found to be associated with increased inflammatory markers.

Maternal stress during pregnancy also affects the gut microbiome of the offspring. Infants born to mothers who reported high stress during pregnancy had less Bifidobacteria, the most important constituent of gut microbiota during infancy and early childhood (Zijlmans et al. 2015). Another study examined the microbiota of teens who lived in an orphanage or foster care during early life (a form of severe early-life stress) and compared it to those raised in stable families. They found that previous adverse care experiences were associated with increased incidence of gastrointestinal symptoms, anxiety, and reduced gut microbiota diversity (Callaghan et al. 2020).

Together, these findings convey that early-life stress adversely affects the gut microbiota, which persists through adolescence and early adulthood. Some of these changes, such as the increased Prevotella abundance, can lead to lifestyle diseases.

Effect of Gut Microbiota on Stress-Response

We learned that stress is characterized by the increased secretion of adrenaline and cortisol. Both these are secreted by the adrenal glands. The process of cortisol secretion starts with the registration of a stressful event by the brain.

It leads to the secretion of Corticotropin-releasing hormone (CRH) from the hypothalamus. CRH stimulates the pituitary gland to secrete ACTH, which stimulates the adrenals to produce cortisol. Thus, the CNS sends a signal to the adrenals in the form of ACTH. This axis is known as the Hypothalamus-pituitary-adrenal (HPA) axis.

Gut microbiota is essential for the development of the HPA axis. It has been proved in an elegant mice study. ACTH and cortisol levels were measured in germ-free and conventionally raised mice. When stressed, both these hormones were higher in germ-free mice compared to the wild mice, suggestive of a heightened stress response. The researchers then enriched the germ-free mice gut with Bifidobacteria and found that the heightened stress response was reversed. The germ-free mice now showed cortisol levels similar to the wild mice in response to stress. The study also found that such reversal of heightened stress response could only be corrected at an early stage, which indicates that gut microbiota is required at an early developmental stage for the HPA axis to become fully susceptible to inhibitory neural signals (Sudo et al. 2004).

In another study, the researchers at Cornell University took two groups of mice – one healthy and the other treated with antibiotics to disrupt the gut microbiota. They put the mice in a chamber where a tone sounded for 30 seconds. When the tone stopped, the mice got an electric shock. The mice started freezing with fear as soon as they heard the tone in anticipation of an electric shock. However, mice can be trained to unlearn such fear. To make them unlearn this fear, the tone was sounded without any shock. After a few sessions of tone without the shock, mice were expected to stop freezing when they heard it. This happened to the normal mice. But the antibiotic-treated group could not stop freezing to the tone long after the shocks had stopped (Chu et al. 2019). To study the mechanism behind this interaction between gut microbiota and stress response, the scientists cut the Vagus nerve in a group of antibiotic-treated mice but it made no difference to the unlearning of fear. They ultimately found that specific gut microbiota metabolites were markedly reduced in the cerebrospinal fluid of the mice who couldn't unlearn the fear. This study showed that the effect of gut microbiota on stress response is mediated primarily via metabolites. In another experimental study, one group of mice was fed SCFAs for one week, and the other group was not. Both the groups underwent three weeks of psychosocial stress. The stress was delivered by keeping the individual mouse with a larger aggressive mouse every day for a specified period. The SCFA fed group had lower levels of stress hormones (cortisol) and showed reduced stress-related behavioral changes compared to the non-SCFA fed group at the end of 3 weeks (Van de Wouw et al. 2018). Again, this study highlights the importance of gut microbiota metabolites, particularly SCFAs, in stress response.

To summarize, the relationship between gut microbiota and stress is bidirectional. Stress has a distinct effect on various body functions. Some of them, such as increased pro-inflammatory markers, are clearly mediated via stress-induced alteration in the gut microbiome. Similarly, the gut microbiome also impacts an individual's stress response which is probably mediated via SCFAs.

Gut Microbiota and Depression

One in five individuals suffers from depression in a lifetime. The gut microbiota composition is altered in individuals with depression. In a large Belgian study, including more than a thousand volunteers, the gut microbiota of depressed individuals was found to lack two specific bacteria, Dialister and Coprococcus, both of which produce butyrate (Valles-Colomer et al. 2019). In another study, Oscillobacter was found to be increased in individuals with depression. Valeric acid, a metabolite produced by Oscillobacter, acts as a natural tranquilizer. Valeric acid mimics the action of GABA, a neurotransmitter that calms the activity in the brain. Increased isovaleric acid levels in stools have been shown to correlate with depression in humans (Szczesniak et al. 2016). Alistipes is another bacterium associated with depression. It interferes with the availability of tryptophan in the intestines. The increased abundance of Alistipes can reduce serotonin levels and lead to depression (Jiang et al. 2015). A recent systematic review of 26 case-control studies found a higher abundance of proinflammatory species (e.g., Enterobacteriaceae) and lower short-chain fatty acid producing bacteria (e.g., Faecalibacterium) in individuals with anxiety and depression (Simpson et al. 2021). Another systematic review published in JAMA showed similar findings with reduced butyrate-producing bacteria *Faecalibacterium* and *Coprococcus* and increased pro-inflammatory bacteria like *Eggerthella* in patients with major depressive disorder, bipolar disorder, psychosis and schizophrenia, and anxiety, suggesting that these disorders are characterized by an alteration in gut microbiota leading to reduction of anti-inflammatory and enrichment of pro-inflammatory genera (Nikolova et al. 2021).

Human trials of probiotics have shown modest benefits in depression. A systematic review showed their benefit in improving the mood in patients with depression (Wallace and Milev, 2017). Another recent meta-analysis, including only RCTs, found that probiotics have a modest effect on depressive symptoms when used as an adjunct to the standard treatment (Nikolova et al. 2019). Many RCTs have been published in the last two years, with the majority showing clinical benefits of probiotics in depression. However, at present, probiotics are not routinely prescribed for the treatment of depression.

Gut Microbiota and Anxiety

Several clinical trials have shown the benefits of probiotics in individuals with anxiety. Two RCTs published in 2019 showed the benefit of long-term (12 to 24 weeks) administration of Lactobacilli in reducing anxiety in healthy individuals who experienced moderate stress. The serum cortisol levels were similar in the Lactobacillus and placebo arms, but pro-inflammatory markers were lesser in the treatment arm (Lew et al. 2019). Sleep quality also improved in the Lactobacillus group (Nishida et al. 2019). However, systematic reviews have not shown much benefit of probiotics in anxiety. A meta-analysis of 23 RCTs showed no significant difference in the symptoms of stress and anxiety between the placebo and probiotic groups (Zagorska et al. 2020). Another systematic review, including young patients (10-24 years), concluded that probiotics have minimal efficacy in the treatment of anxiety (Cohen et al. 2021). Another meta-analysis, including 30 RCTs, did not show any qualitative benefit of probiotics in stress and anxiety (Le Morvan et al. 2022). Probiotics are not recommended for anxiety treatment in routine clinical practice.

Current Practice

Probiotics

They are not recommended to treat stress-related disorders in routine clinical practice. They are the most common microbiota therapy studied in clinical trials, but the benefits are not yet conclusively proven.

FMT: Clinical trials are lacking in the treatment of anxiety and depression. It may prove to be more effective than probiotics.

Chapter 7

Gut Microbiota: Role in Gastrointestinal Disorders

Goals

1. To know about the role of gut microbiota in the pathophysiology of irritable bowel syndrome.
2. To know about the role of gut microbiota in inflammatory bowel disease
3. To know the clinical applications

By now, it is obvious that gut microbiota plays a role in gastrointestinal diseases. Studies have established its role in irritable bowel syndrome (IBS), inflammatory bowel diseases (IBD), alcoholic liver diseases, non-alcoholic fatty liver disease (NAFLD), cirrhosis, *Clostridium difficile* infection, and colorectal cancer. We shall discuss only the IBS and IBD in this chapter.

Gut Microbiota and Irritable Bowel Syndrome (IBS)

IBS is characterized by abdominal pain related to defecation and is associated with a change in stool form or frequency. It is recognized as a disorder of brain-gut interaction. The pathophysiology of IBS is multifactorial. A number of factors, including GI motility, visceral hypersensitivity or increased visceral pain perception, gut dysbiosis, GI infections, altered central pain pathways, immune dysfunction, and mucosal inflammation, are implicated in IBS development. The gut microbiota plays a role in many of these factors.

According to Rome IV criteria, IBS is diagnosed if a person has recurrent abdominal pain, on average at least one day per week during the previous three months, with two or more of the following:

1. Related to defecation
2. Associated with a change in stool frequency
3. Associated with a change in stool form

IBS is further divided into four subtypes based on stool form. They are diarrhea-predominant (IBS-D), constipation-predominant (IBS-C),) mixed (IBS-M) and unsubtyped (IBS-U).

Biological Plausibility

Alteration in gut microbiota leads to increased visceral pain perception and low-grade mucosal inflammation. This is supported by the development of post-infectious IBS. In post-infectious IBS, after an acute GI infection is cured, the symptoms persist and may last even for several months. The GI infection is controlled, but the ensuing visceral hypersensitivity leads to the development of symptoms. The presence of the microbiome-gut-brain axis, too, is an indicator of the role of gut microbiota in IBS, which is a disorder of brain-gut interaction.

Evidence from Animal Studies

The germ-free mice have increased visceral pain perception, which gets reversed when they are colonized by the gut microbiota from conventionally raised mice (Luczynsk et al 2017). They also show central nervous system alterations, mainly in the form of reduced volume of the anterior cingulate cortex, which is a pain-processing site, suggesting that gut microbiota may be involved in the development of central pain-processing pathways.

Alteration of mice gut microbiota by antibiotics in early life has been shown to result in a long-lasting increase in visceral pain. Treatment with vancomycin in early life led to increased visceral pain as measured by balloon rectal distension in adult mice (O'Mahony et al. 2014). In another mice study, early-life stress induced by separation from the mother also led to increased visceral pain and reduced fecal microbiota diversity. The administration of probiotic bacteria Faecalibacterium prausnazii reduced the visceral pain in these mice (Miquel et al. 2016).

In an interesting study, fecal microbiota from constipation-predominant IBS patients and healthy individuals were transplanted into two groups of mice. It led to increased visceral hypersensitivity in the group transplanted with IBS microbiota, whereas the other group remained normal (Crouzet et al. 2013). This study provides direct evidence of the role of gut microbiota in the increased visceral pain perception or visceral hypersensitivity.

Gut microbiota dysbiosis results in increased mucosal and systemic inflammation, as already discussed in chapter 4. Low dose injections of bacterial lipopolysaccharide (LPS) in mice have been shown to trigger rectal pain sensation (Nozu et al. 2017). Another mice study, in which mucosal inflammation was induced chemically, found that if the inflammation is severe, the subsequent visceral hypersensitivity is also severe (Adam et al. 2006). These studies indicate a link between dysbiosis, mucosal inflammation, and visceral hypersensitivity (Figure 7.1). Gut microbiota's role in immune development and function is discussed in chapter 3.

To summarize, animal studies provide insights into the role of gut microbiota in various pathophysiological mechanisms responsible for the development of symptoms in IBS.

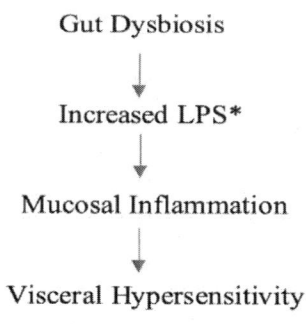

*LPS, Lipopolysaccharide.

Figure 7.1. Role of gut microbiota in the development of IBS.

Evidence from Human Studies

The gut microbiota of individuals with IBS differs from those without IBS. A review published in the journal Nature in 2014 concluded that IBS patients have gut dysbiosis, primarily in the form of reduced microbial diversity. The alteration in gut microbiota is more pronounced in patients with IBS-D (Collins SM 2014). However, there was no specific bacterial genus or species which could be identified as a microbial marker or signature of IBS.

A study published in 2018 found Faecalibacterium to be reduced in patients with IBS-D (Maharashak et al. 2018), while another study found Bacteroides to be increased in IBS-D and Bifidobacteria to be reduced in both IBS-D and IBS-C (Fredericks et al. 2020). A study in preadolescent children

(7 to 12 years) found differences in gut microbiota, gene functions, and metabolites between children with IBS and healthy controls (Hollister et al. 2019). Flavonifractor plautii and Lachnospiraceae were increased in children with IBS. Fecal secondary bile acids were elevated in the children with IBS, and their levels correlated with the severity of abdominal pain, as were the fecal cholesterol levels, which correlated with the frequency of abdominal pain.

A meta-analysis that included both RCTs and case-control studies found SCFAs to be altered in patients with IBS. In IBS-C patients, propionate and butyrate were reduced, whereas butyrate was increased in IBS-D patients compared to healthy controls (Sun et al. 2019).

Clinical Trials

Various studies have shown microbiota therapy to be beneficial in individuals with IBS. A meta-analysis published as early as 2011 showed the benefit of probiotic Lactobacillus rhamnosus for the treatment of abdominal pain in children with IBS and functional GI disorders (Horvath et al. 2011). Another meta-analysis in 2014 showed the benefits of probiotics on abdominal pain, bloating, and flatulence in patients with IBS (Ford et al. 2014). However, an RCT evaluating Bifidobacterium infantis in 275 IBS patients did not find any improvement in abdominal pain or bloating (Ringel-Kulka et al. 2017).

A large meta-analysis including 53 RCTs and 5545 patients found that certain probiotic combinations and specific specie or strains had beneficial effects on global IBS symptoms and abdominal pain but concluded that their efficacy could not be definitively proven. It also found an antibiotic, rifaximin, to be effective in patients with non-constipation predominant IBS (Ford et al. 2018).

Due to such discrepancies in findings, American Gastroenterology Association (AGA) conducted a technical review on the efficacy of probiotics in IBS. It reviewed the literature from inception till December 2018 and included a collective of 5301 subjects and 44 different probiotic formulations. It concluded that the overall certainty of the evidence for the use of probiotics to treat IBS is low (Preidis et al. 2020). The AGA guidelines acknowledge the current knowledge gaps and recommend using probiotics only in clinical trials. Prebiotics and synbiotics are also studied for the treatment of IBS with varied results but, until now, are not recommended by the guidelines for routine clinical use.

FMT has also been evaluated as the microbiome-based therapy in IBS. An RCT in 2018 showed the benefit of FMT in patients with moderate to severe IBS. 65% of patients in the FMT group showed improvement as compared to 43% in the placebo group (Johnsen et al. 2018). However, another RCT using oral capsules (containing freeze-dried donor stools) as the mode of FMT did not show any benefit (Aroniadis et al. 2019). A meta-analysis published in 2019 found that FMT did not improve symptoms in IBS. It noted that most of the FMT studies were conducted in IBS-D or IBS-M patients, with only 9% of patients belonging to the IBS-C subtype. However, it showed that FMT delivered through colonoscopy had benefits, but the oral capsules were ineffective (Xu et al. 2019).

The benefit of FMT in IBS is shown to be mediated via SCFAs. The fecal analysis of patients recruited in an RCT which showed the benefit of FMT found that butyrate levels increased significantly after FMT and correlated with the improvement in IBS symptoms (El-Salhy et al. 2021). The latest meta-analysis published in 2022 found that FMT delivered via colonoscopy or gastroscopy was superior to placebo, but the oral FMT capsules were not. One year after the application, the benefits of FMT were absent (Wu et al. 2022).

To summarize, human studies show that gut microbiota is altered in IBS, particularly IBS-D. In the form of probiotics, microbiota therapy has shown benefits in abdominal pain and global IBS symptoms. FMT is effective only when delivered via gastroscopy or colonoscopy. However, more robust evidence is needed to recommend these for routine clinical use.

Current Practice

Probiotics can be used to relieve abdominal pain and global symptoms in IBS as per the British Society of Gastroenterology guidelines (Vasant et al. 2021). Although, it is a weak recommendation with low-quality evidence. American College of Gastroenterology recommends against the use of probiotics in IBS.

FMT is currently recommended only in the setting of clinical trials in IBS.

Gut Microbiota and Inflammatory Bowel Disease (IBD)

IBD is characterized by the development of an abnormal immune response against a subset of commensal intestinal bacteria in genetically predisposed individuals leading to a state of chronic inflammation and injury (Ramos & Papadakis 2019). IBD phenotypically is divided into two major forms, ulcerative colitis and Crohn's disease. We shall not go into the details of these phenotypes, and for the purpose of this discussion, I shall refer to IBD as a single entity.

Biological Plausibility

The intestinal microbiota plays a central role in the development of IBD. Diversion of the fecal stream by the surgical ileostomy leads to a dramatic response in patients with IBD, highlighting that the gut microbial antigens are necessary to activate immune response and inflammation. Besides, the gut microbiota is essential for developing the gastrointestinal immune system, as discussed in chapter 3. The various pathophysiological mechanisms for the development of IBD and their possible relation to gut microbiota are outlined in Table 7.1.

Table 7.1. Pathophysiology of IBD and the role of gut microbiota

	Mechanism of IBD development	Possible preventive role of Gut microbiota
1.	Abnormal immune response	Helps in the development of tolerance by increasing IL-10 and TGF-β and differentiation and expansion of T regs.
2.	Impaired microbial antigens recognition and clearance by the innate immune system	Helps in the development and maturation of the innate immune system.
3.	Persistence of mucosal inflammation	Produces metabolites like SCFAs, which have anti-inflammatory properties.
4.	Poor healing of tissue injury	Promotes tissue healing by stimulating mucous production.

The gut microbiota in IBD is characterized by the following alterations:

1. Reduced gut microbial diversity, primarily the Firmicutes. Firmicutes are the prime fermenters of the complex carbohydrates leading to the production of SCFAs, which have anti-inflammatory properties. Clostridiales and Faecalibacterium prausnitzzi are particularly reduced in the intestinal microbiota in IBD.

2. Increased abundance of mucolytic bacteria, e.g., Ruminococcus gnavas. The mucous layer in the human intestines is an essential component of the intestinal barrier. It prevents the interaction between the intestinal epithelium and microbial antigens and also promotes healing of the epithelium after injury. The damage to the mucous layer thus leads to increased chances of immune activation and persistent tissue injury.
3. Increase in sulfate-reducing bacteria such as desulfovibrio in ulcerative colitis. Increased sulfate reduction leads to the production of hydrogen sulfate which damages the intestinal barrier.
4. Increased abundance of proteobacteria, which are associated with mucosal and systemic inflammation, particularly an increase in enteroadhesive E. coli.

Evidence from Scientific Studies

Various scientific studies have demonstrated gut microbiota alteration in patients with IBD, primarily in the form of reduced microbial diversity (Pittayanon et al. 2020). There is a reduced abundance of bacteria with anti-inflammatory properties and an increase in bacteria with pro-inflammatory properties. Six of the eleven studies of Faecalibacterium prausnitzii in IBD reported a decreased abundance as compared to controls, whereas two different studies of E. coli in Crohn's disease reported its increased abundance. At the taxonomic level of phyla, the studies have reported a reduction in Firmicutes and an increase in Proteobacteria (Nishida et al. 2018). E. coli is found to be increased up to 10 times in the ileum of patients with ileal Crohn's disease (Darfeuille-Michaud & Colombel 2008).

Mucolytic bacteria are characterized by the ability to degrade human secretory mucin. They are shown to be increased, even in histologically normal mucosa, in patients with both ulcerative colitis and Crohn's disease (Png et al. 2010). The damage to the mucous layer leads to increased immune activation and poor tissue healing, the hallmark features of IBD.

The number of short-chain fatty acids producing bacteria (eg. Faecalibacterium prausnitzzi) gets reduced in IBD, affecting the differentiation and expansion of T regs which are the chief cells that limit the activation of the gut immune system. A meta-analysis evaluating the case-control studies on SCFAs in IBD found each of the acetate, propionate, and butyrate to be reduced in patients with ulcerative colitis and Crohn's disease

(Zhuang et al. 2019). Another systematic review, including metabolomic studies in IBD, found gut microbial metabolites such as secondary bile acids to be reduced in the stools of IBD patients (Gallagher et al. 2021).

Clinical Trials

Probiotics have been studied extensively in patients with IBD and have shown benefits in ulcerative colitis but not in Crohn's disease. As early as 2005, 6-week treatment with VSL-3, a multi-strain probiotic, showed benefit in mild to moderately severe ulcerative colitis (Bibiloni et al. 2005). A meta-analysis including only the RCTs found that VSL-3 showed benefit in UC in the induction as well as maintenance of remission while other probiotic formulations were not better than placebo. No benefit of probiotics was found in Crohn's disease (Derwa et al. 2017). Another meta-analysis, including RCTs of probiotics in Crohn's disease, did not find them to be beneficial (Limetkai et al. 2020). Another one published in 2021 found that probiotics and synbiotic supplements based on Lactobacillus and Bifidobacterium or more than one strain, such as VSL-3, were beneficial in UC (Zhang et al. 2021).

The other microbiota therapy studied in patients with IBD is FMT, including both the oral capsules and colonoscopically or enteral tubes delivered FMT. An early meta-analysis published in 2014, including 18 studies though only one RCT, found FMT to be efficacious both in UC and Crohn's disease (Colman & Rubin 2014). In an RCT of weekly FMT given for six weeks, 24 % of UC patients achieved clinical remission compared to 5% on placebo. Stools of patients receiving FMT had greater microbial diversity compared with baseline than that of patients who received placebo (Moayyedi et al. 2015).

A meta-analysis published in 2017, including 53 studies, again found FMT to be effective in IBD. 50% of Crohn's disease and 36% of UC patients achieved clinical remission. FMT also increased the diversity of the recipients' gut microbiota (Paramsothy et al. 2017). However, another meta-analysis, including only the high-quality RCTs, noted that no eligible study was available for FMT in Crohn's disease (Imdad et al. 2018). Since then, 2 RCTs have been published studying the role of FMT in Crohn's disease. FMT was found to be beneficial as compared to placebo, both in the induction of clinical remission (67 % of patients) (Yang et al. 2020) and maintenance of steroid-free remission (87 % of patients at week 10) (Sokol et al. 2020). However, the number of patients in each trial was small, 27 and 17, respectively. To conclude, FMT is shown to benefit around one-third of ulcerative colitis and one-half to two-thirds of Crohn's disease patients. However, good quality RCTs with a large number of patients are lacking, especially in Crohn's disease.

Current Practice

Both probiotics and FMT are not recommended as routine treatments for either ulcerative colitis or Crohn's disease (Raine et al. 2022, Torres et al. 2020). Currently, they can be used in the setting of clinical trials only.

Chapter 8

The Microbiota Therapies

Goals

1. To know about the various methods of administration of microbiota therapy
2. To know various terminologies like prebiotics, probiotics, synbiotics, postbiotics, etc.
3. To know about fecal microbiota transplantation
4. To know about the scientific evidence for the use of microbiota therapy

The 'microbiota therapies' or 'microbiome-based therapies' are the means to alter the microbiome of an individual in such a way as to deliver health benefits. If the gut microbes impact a large number of physiological functions in our body and are altered in various disease states, they can also be harnessed to improve health and cure illnesses.

There are many ways to deliver microbiota therapy:

1. *Diet:* Diet is the foremost factor that influences the gut microbiome. A high-fiber diet rich in complex carbohydrates leads to an increased abundance of Firmicutes and elevated SCFA production. Another dietary way to alter the gut microbiota is fermented foods. Fermented foods like curd, miso, kefir, kanji, kimchi, sauerkraut, etc., are rich in beneficial bacteria or fungi. Their regular consumption provides these to the recipient and alters their gut microbiome.
2. *Prebiotics:* Prebiotics are the compounds utilized by gut microbes. We shall learn the precise definition of prebiotics soon. If bacteria are the plants in the garden of the intestines, then prebiotics are manure. Prebiotics alter the gut microbiota by providing the raw materials for the growth of beneficial bacteria in the intestines. The next set of microbiota therapies relies on delivering the microbes themselves to the human intestines.

3. *Probiotics:* Probiotics are the live beneficial microbes given orally in capsules, powders, liquids, etc., in large quantities to alter the gut microbiota. They, like prebiotics, are also precisely defined, which we shall learn soon.
4. *Synbiotics*: Synbiotics are the combination of prebiotics and probiotics.
5. *Fecal Microbiota Transplant (FMT):* FMT is perhaps the most ingenious way to deliver the gut microbiota to a recipient. In FMT, the stools from a suitable healthy donor are administered to the recipient via colonoscopy or enteral tubes. It can deliver a huge amount and a larger variety of microbes than probiotics. In FMT, the gut microbiota of a diseased recipient is replaced by the healthy microbiota of the donor, possibly leading to the disease cure.
6. Postbiotics: Postbiotics are the new entrants to the gamut of microbiota therapy. They are dead or inanimate microbes in contrast to the probiotics which are living micro-organisms.

Prebiotics

As per the International Scientific Association for Probiotics and Prebiotics (ISAPP), a prebiotic is defined as a substrate that is selectively utilized by host microorganisms conferring a health benefit (Gibson et al. 2017). The terms fiber, microbiota accessible carbohydrates (MACs), and prebiotics are often used interchangeably, but there is a subtle difference between them.

Fibers are complex carbohydrates that are not digested by human digestive enzymes. Not all the undigested dietary fiber is utilized by the intestinal microbes. Only those fiber or complex carbohydrates that are used by the microbiota are called microbiota accessible carbohydrates or MACs. Thus, all fibers are not MACs.

Prebiotics are precisely defined and must confer a proven health benefit to the recipient. Thus, the compounds scientifically studied and proven to provide a health benefit are termed prebiotics. Prebiotics also include compounds other than carbohydrates, such as polyphenols. Similarly, only those MACs which provide a proven health benefit are prebiotics.

A wide range of plant-based foods provides prebiotics, both in the form of MACs and polyphenols. Prebiotics are also available as food supplements and tablets e.g., Inulin tablets. Prebiotics have been studied for various illnesses such as IBS and obesity, alone and in combination with probiotics but are not currently recommended as the routine treatment by the scientific guidelines.

Probiotics

Probiotics are defined as 'live microorganisms that, when administered in adequate amounts, confer a health benefit on the host.'

They can either be consumed as fermented foods, which are a rich source of beneficial bacteria, or as probiotic supplements. Probiotic supplements are available in a varied range of products such as tablets, capsules, sachets, and liquid formulations. The probiotic VSL#3[1] is one of the most commonly prescribed probiotics. It contains eight different strains of bacteria, including four strains of Lactobacilli, three strains of Bifidobacteria, and *Streptococcus thermophiles*. It is available as sachets and capsules and contains 900 billion live bacteria in the highest dose packaging. It appears to be a large number, but these many bacteria are present in just 1 ml of colonic content.

There are many challenges to the use of probiotics as microbiota therapy. These include:

1. *Cost:* Probiotics are live bacteria. Providing them in the form of capsules, sachets, etc. is expensive.
2. *Fragility:* Probiotics are fragile. They must survive the process of manufacturing, supplies, and storage, and also the gastric acid and digestive enzymes.
3. *Regulatory indecisiveness:* Probiotics are categorized by most of the regulatory authorities, including the FDA, as dietary supplements and not as medicines that are subject to stricter controls. This allows for a wide difference in the number and strains of bacteria in the probiotic supplements. Though most of the leading formulations contain 5-20 billion live bacteria per serving, there are large differences. Similarly, both single strain and multi-strain probiotics are available.

Despite the challenges, probiotics are the most preferred form of microbiota therapy. Their availability, ease of administration, and wide acceptability make them the first choice agents for delivering beneficial microbes to patients. They are routinely prescribed and have a proven role in

---

[1] VSL#3 is now available as visbiome worldwide.

irritable bowel syndrome (Ford et al. 2014), ileal pouch inflammation (pouchitis) (Nguyen et al. 2019), and prevention of antibiotic-associated diarrhea (Goldenberg et al. 2019). Besides, they are also being studied with mixed results in a wide range of illnesses, as mentioned in earlier chapters. Probiotic supplements with newer microbial species and strains are being constantly developed. With the advent of the newer formulations and expansion of their usage, probiotics are going to remain the foremost tool to alter the gut microbiome

'Psychobiotics' are a special class of probiotics. They are the live microorganisms that, when administered in adequate amounts, confer a mental health benefit to the host. They influence the microbiome-brain-gut interaction. The various possible mechanisms and the impact of gut microbiota on stress and related disorders and the scientific evidence on the use of probiotics/psychobiotics in mental health disorders are described in chapter 6.

'Next generation probiotics (NGP)' are a new exciting tool in the gamut of microbiota therapy. They are newly isolated gut bacteria that have beneficial properties. Besides naturally occurring commensals, NGPs also include genetically modified bacteria designed to provide health benefits to recipients. NGPs differ from traditional probiotics, primarily in their clinical application. While conventional probiotics are being used to improve overall health and in a wide variety of diseases, the NGPs are specifically targeted against a particular disease. NGPs are shown to have both preventive as well as therapeutic applications (Chang et al. 2019). They include various bacteria like:

Christensenella minuta (phylum Firmicutes): This bacterium is shown to be associated with a reduction in obesity and metabolic syndrome and produces large amounts of acetate and butyrate. Invitro studies using human intestinal cell lines have shown it to have strong anti-inflammatory properties by inhibiting NF-κB signaling (Kropp C et al. 2021).

Akkermansia muciniphila (phylum Verrucomicrobia): It resides in the intestinal mucous layer. Pasteurized *A. muciniphila* has been shown to prevent the development of obesity and insulin resistance in mice. A purified membrane protein (Amuc_1100) is responsible for the beneficial effects of the bacterium (Plovier et al. 2017).

Faecalibacterium prausnitzii (phylum Firmicutes): It also has anti-inflammatory properties and improves the gut barrier function (Xiaoya et al. 2021).

Lots of other bacteria are being studied as possible NGPs. Most are currently in the nascent stage of development, with only animal studies showing beneficial effects. But, if NGPs are found to provide clinically meaningful benefits in humans, they will change the treatment of many diseases in the future.

Fecal Microbiota Transplant (FMT)

FMT, surprisingly, is the oldest form of microbiota therapy. It has been described in Chinese medicine as early as the 4th century AD. In modern medicine, FMT was first reported in 1958 in patients with pseudomembranous enterocolitis (Eiseman et al. 1958).

The FMT is the process of the transfer of gut microbiota from a healthy donor to a diseased recipient. It is achieved by transplanting the feces from the donor to the recipient, thus termed fecal microbiota transplant (FMT). It is done by colonoscopy, in which liquid slurry prepared of the donor feces is instilled into the recipient's colon directly. The liquid slurry is usually infused in 50 to 60 ml aliquots over the colonic walls, starting from the caecum up to the mid-transverse colon. The process, however, differs considerably based on the patient's condition and the practices of the treating team. The entire slurry (usually 200 ml to 500 ml) can also be safely instilled in the right colon as it gets transferred across the whole colon by peristalsis. The recipient is encouraged to hold the stools for at least 2 hours after the procedure. FMT can also be applied by enema, which is less invasive and costly, and particularly useful in critically ill patients, but is less efficacious and may require multiple sessions (Cammarota et al. 2017).

FMT is also performed via the upper GI tract. The fecal slurry is delivered through the gastroscope or enteral tubes and the recipient is kept in a 45° upright position for 4 hours to prevent aspiration.

FMT is also done with frozen stools. The stools are frozen at -80 °C and thawed on the day of the process and instilled within 6 hours of preparation. The frozen stool FMT is promising for the future development of stool banks, which will obviate the need to identify a suitable donor and provide timely therapy to the patients. The frozen and fresh stools have equal treatment efficacy in patients with recurrent *C. difficile* infection (Lee et al. 2016).

But, the latest and the most acceptable method (to the recipient) of FMT is the oral capsule. It utilizes the stool mixed with a cryoprotectant such as glycerol. The stool is centrifuged, the supernatant is discarded, and the sediment is filled in capsules and flash frozen on dry ice. The capsules are stored at -70° C and used when required. Studies have shown the oral capsules to be equally effective as the colonoscope delivered fecal transplants in *C. difficile* infection (Kao et al. 2017). The definite advantages of capsule FMT are patient acceptability, ease of application, and non-requirement of identifying donors, but the number of microbes provided is smaller than colonoscopic FMT.

The most crucial aspect of FMT is donor screening. Stool donors undergo an exhaustive preliminary evaluation, followed by blood and stool investigations. The donors are asked about the usage of antibiotics, chemotherapy, immunosuppressant drugs, and long-term proton pump inhibitors over the last three months. They also inform about the history of any chronic gastrointestinal disease, gastrointestinal cancers, autoimmune disorders, known blood-borne infections such as hepatitis B, hepatitis C, HIV, HTLV I and II, obesity, neurobehavioral conditions, high-risk behavior, illicit drug use, needle stick injury, body piercing, tattooing, acupuncture in the last six months, recent acute gastroenteritis, and vaccination with any live vaccine (Bibbò et al. 2020). They undergo various blood and stool investigations, summarized in Table 8.1. Donors are rigorously screened to select the ones with healthy gut microbiota and to prevent the transmission of diseases. Though mostly the FMT is done with donor stools, autologous FMT using the patient's own stools is also reported. In inflammatory bowel diseases, patients' stools collected during remission have been used during the relapse (Duplessis et al. 2012).

The prime advantage of FMT is that it provides a much larger number and variety of gut microbes as compared to other forms of microbiota therapy such as probiotics. The disadvantages include poor widespread acceptability, the requirement of invasive procedures, donor screening, and cost. There remains a risk of transmission of drug-resistant pathogens despite the exhaustive donor screening. Recently, a report described two patients who developed extended-spectrum beta-lactamase-producing *Escherichia coli* bacteremia after FMT (De Fillip et al. 2019). The development of frozen stool banks and capsule FMT can overcome some of these limitations and establish FMT as a prime treatment for many diseases.

FMT is studied in a large number of diseases. A glance at *ClinicalTrials.gov,* a database of all the clinical trials, shows that more than 90 FMT trials in a myriad of conditions ranging from liver failure, metabolic syndrome, and cancers to neurological disorders are currently recruiting subjects.

But it is the first-line treatment only for recurrent *Clostridium difficile* infection. It has shown promising results in inflammatory bowel diseases

(Paramsothy et al. 2017) and IBS (Johnsen et al. 2019) but is not used routinely in these patients.

Postbiotics

The recent observation that 'some health benefits of probiotics are not dependent on their viability' has led to the development of the concept of postbiotics. The health benefits of many fermented foods which are traditionally consumed after cooking and thus do not contain live bacteria are presumably due to the effects of postbiotics.

Postbiotics are defined by the International Scientific Association for Probiotics and Prebiotics (ISAPP) as a "preparation of inanimate microorganisms and/or their components that confers a health benefit on the host (Salminen et al. 2021)." In other words, postbiotics are non-viable microbes (whole or cell components) with or without microbial metabolites. Their most significant advantage is that they make the viability of bacteria non-essential for health benefits, which can increase the accessibility and reduce the cost of postbiotic formations compared to probiotics.

The following preparations are not considered postbiotics:

1. Vaccines
2. Filtrates without cell components
3. Purified microbial components and metabolites (For e.g., Purified preparation of SCFAs or other organic acids)

Microbial components are essential for a formulation to be labeled as postbiotic. A postbiotic is not simply a dead probiotic bacterium. It may be a completely different strain or specie which has no proven role as a probiotic. Postbiotics are also used for applications at sites other than the gut. Postbiotic oral lozenges of Lactobacillus salivarius and L. paracasei have been shown to improve oral hygiene, reduce pathogens, and increase the beneficial bacteria in the oral cavity (Lin et al. 2022).

There are various possible mechanisms for the health benefits of postbiotics. Metabolites such as SCFAs, neurotransmitters, and microbial enzymes in postbiotic preparations are one of the prime reasons for their efficacy. The dead microbes in the postbiotics express adhesion molecules that can compete with the intestinal microbiota for colonization. They also express PAMPs and thus can modulate the local and systemic immune response.

Few scientific studies on postbiotics have been done due to their recent development. They are being studied both in animals and humans. An oral Lactobacillus rhamnosus postbiotic has been shown to be effective in children with atopic dermatitis, reducing the symptoms and inflammatory markers (Jeong et al. 2020). An anti-regurgitation formula containing postbiotics along with fructo and galactooligosaccharides was found to reduce the GI symptoms in formula-fed infants with regurgitation (Bellaiche et al. 2021). And lastly, a systematic review of 7 RCTs showed postbiotic Lactobacillus acidophilus to be effective in the treatment and L. paracasei in the prevention of diarrhea in children (Malagón-Rojas et al. 2020). However, the RCTs were all done before 2020, while the consensus definition of postbiotics was finalized in 2021. Thus, future studies with rigorously identified postbiotics will shed further light on their efficacy in human disease.

This brings us to the end of this chapter on microbiota or microbiome-based therapies. They are promising, with newer modes of delivery and microbial strains being developed rapidly. They stand on a sound base of all we have learned in this book but are clinically useful in only a small number of diseases at present.

Bibliography

Chapter 1

Allen, J. M., Mailing, L. J., Niemiro, G. M., Moore, R., Cook, M. D., White, B. A., Holscher, H. D., & Woods, J. A. 2018. Exercise Alters Gut Microbiota Composition and Function in Lean and Obese Humans. *Medicine and science in sports and exercise*, *50*: 747–57. https://doi.org/10.1249/MSS.0000000000001495.

Arumugam, M., Raes, J., Pelletier, E., Le Paslier, D., Yamada, T., Mende, D. R., Fernandes, G. R., Tap, J., Bruls, T., Batto, J. M., Bertalan, M., Borruel, N., Casellas, F., Fernandez, L., Gautier, L., Hansen, T., Hattori, M., Hayashi, T., Kleerebezem, M., Kurokawa, K., Bork, P. 2011. Enterotypes of the human gut microbiome. *Nature*, *473*, 174–180. https://doi.org/10.1038/nature09944.

Azevedo, M. J., Pereira, M. L., Araujo, R., Ramalho, C., Zaura, E., & Sampaio-Maia, B. 2020. Influence of delivery and feeding mode in oral fungi colonization - a systematic review. *Microbial cell (Graz, Austria)*, *7*, 36–45. https://doi.org/10.15698/mic2020.02.706.

Barber, C., Mego, M., Sabater, C., Vallejo, F., Bendezu, R. A., Masihy, M., Guarner, F., Espín, J. C., Margolles, A., & Azpiroz, F. 2021. Differential Effects of Western and Mediterranean-Type Diets on Gut Microbiota: A Metagenomics and Metabolomics Approach. *Nutrients*, *13*, 2638. https://doi.org/10.3390/nu13082638.

Benedict, C., Vogel, H., Jonas, W., Woting, A., Blaut, M., Schürmann, A., &Cedernaes, J. 2016. Gut microbiota and glucometabolic alterations in response to recurrent partial sleep deprivation in normal-weight young individuals. *Molecular metabolism*, *5*(12): 1175–86. https://doi.org/10.1016/j.molmet.2016.10.003

Bezirtzoglou, E., Tsiotsias, A., & Welling, G. W. 2011. Microbiota profile in feces of breast- and formula-fed newborns by using fluorescence in situ hybridization (FISH). *Anaerobe*, *17*(6): 478–82. https://doi.org/10.1016/j.anaerobe.2011.03.009

Braden T. Tierney, Zhen Yang, Jacob M. Luber, Marc Beaudin, Marsha C. Wibowo, Christina Baek, Eleanor Mehlenbacher, Chirag J. Patel, Aleksandar D. Kostic.2019. The Landscape of Genetic Content in the Gut and Oral Human Microbiome. *Cell Host & Microbe*, *26*: 283 doi: 10.1016/j.chom.2019.07.008.

Chambers, E. S., Byrne, C. S., Morrison, D. J., Murphy, K. G., Preston, T., Tedford, C., Garcia-Perez, I., Fountana, S., Serrano-Contreras, J. I., Holmes, E., Reynolds, C. J., Roberts, J. F., Boyton, R. J., Altmann, D. M., McDonald, J., Marchesi, J. R., Akbar, A. N., Riddell, N. E., Wallis, G. A., & Frost, G. S. 2019. Dietary supplementation with inulin-propionate ester or inulin improves insulin sensitivity in adults with overweight and obesity with distinct effects on the gut microbiota, plasma metabolome and systemic inflammatory responses: a randomised cross-over trial. *Gut*, *68*, 1430–1438. https://doi.org/10.1136/gutjnl-2019-318424.

Clarke, S. F., Murphy, E. F., O'Sullivan, O., Lucey, A. J., Humphreys, M., Hogan, A., Hayes, P., O'Reilly, M., Jeffery, I. B., Wood-Martin, R., Kerins, D. M., Quigley, E., Ross, R. P., O'Toole, P. W., Molloy, M. G., Falvey, E., Shanahan, F., & Cotter, P. D.

2014. Exercise and associated dietary extremes impact on gut microbial diversity. *Gut*, *63*:1913–20. https://doi.org/10.1136/gutjnl-2013-306541.

Coker, O. O., Nakatsu, G., Dai, R. Z., Wu, W., Wong, S. H., Ng, S. C., Chan, F., Sung, J., & Yu, J. 2019. Enteric fungal microbiota dysbiosis and ecological alterations in colorectal cancer. *Gut*, *68*, 654–662. https://doi.org/10.1136/gutjnl-2018-317178.

Costantini, L., Molinari, R., Farinon, B., & Merendino, N. 2017. Impact of Omega-3 Fatty Acids on the Gut Microbiota. International journal of molecular sciences, 18: 2645. https://doi.org/10.3390/ijms18122645.

De Filippis, F., Pellegrini, N., Vannini, L., Jeffery, I. B., La Storia, A., Laghi, L., Serrazanetti, D. I., Di Cagno, R., Ferrocino, I., Lazzi, C., Turroni, S., Cocolin, L., Brigidi, P., Neviani, E., Gobbetti, M., O'Toole, P. W., &Ercolini, D. 2016. High-level adherence to a Mediterranean diet beneficially impacts the gut microbiota and associated metabolome. *Gut*, *65*:1812–21. https://doi.org/10.1136/gutjnl-2015-309957.

Deaver, J. A., Eum, S. Y., &Toborek, M. 2018. Circadian Disruption Changes Gut Microbiome Taxa and Functional Gene Composition. *Frontiers in microbiology*, *9*, 737. https://doi.org/10.3389/fmicb.2018.00737.

Dhakan, D. B., Maji, A., Sharma, A. K., Saxena, R., Pulikkan, J., Grace, T., Gomez, A., Scaria, J., Amato, K. R., & Sharma, V. K. 2019. The unique composition of Indian gut microbiome, gene catalogue, and associated fecalmetabolome deciphered using multi-omics approaches. *GigaScience*, 8: giz004. https://doi.org/10.1093/gigascience/giz004.

Dominguez-Bello, M. G., Costello, E. K., Contreras, M., Magris, M., Hidalgo, G., Fierer, N., & Knight, R. 2010. Delivery mode shapes the acquisition and structure of the initial microbiota across multiple body habitats in newborns. *Proceedings of the National Academy of Sciences of the United States of America*, *107*: 11971–5. https://doi.org/10.1073/pnas.1002601107.

Dong, T. S., Luu, K., Lagishetty, V., Sedighian, F., Woo, S. L., Dreskin, B. W., Katzka, W., Chang, C., Zhou, Y., Arias-Jayo, N., Yang, J., Ahdoot, A., Li, Z., Pisegna, J. R., & Jacobs, J. P. 2020. A High Protein Calorie Restriction Diet Alters the Gut Microbiome in Obesity. *Nutrients*, *12*, 3221. https://doi.org/10.3390/nu12103221.

Estaki, M., Pither, J., Baumeister, P., Little, J. P., Gill, S. K., Ghosh, S., Ahmadi-Vand, Z., Marsden, K. R., & Gibson, D. L. 2016. Cardiorespiratory fitness as a predictor of intestinal microbial diversity and distinct metagenomic functions. *Microbiome*, *4*, 42. https://doi.org/10.1186/s40168-016-0189-7.

Galazzo, G., van Best, N., Bervoets, L., Dapaah, I. O., Savelkoul, P. H., Hornef, M. W., GI-MDH consortium, Lau, S., Hamelmann, E., &Penders, J. 2020. Development of the Microbiota and Associations With Birth Mode, Diet, and Atopic Disorders in a Longitudinal Analysis of Stool Samples, Collected From Infancy Through Early Childhood. *Gastroenterology*, *158*: 1584–96. https://doi.org/10.1053/j.gastro.2020.01.024.

Huang, H., Krishnan, H. B., Pham, Q., Yu, L. L., & Wang, T. T. 2016. Soy and Gut Microbiota: Interaction and Implication for Human Health. *Journal of agricultural and food chemistry*, 64, 8695–8709. https://doi.org/10.1021/acs.jafc.6b03725.

Bibliography

Imhann, F., Bonder, M. J., Vich Vila, A., Fu, J., Mujagic, Z., Vork, L., Tigchelaar, E. F., Jankipersadsing, S. A., Cenit, M. C., Harmsen, H. J., Dijkstra, G., Franke, L., Xavier, R. J., Jonkers, D., Wijmenga, C., Weersma, R. K., &Zhernakova, A. 2016. Proton pump inhibitors affect the gut microbiome. *Gut*, *65*: 740–8. https://doi.org/10.1136/gutjnl-2015-310376.

Jain, U., Ver Heul, A. M., Xiong, S., Gregory, M. H., Demers, E. G., Kern, J. T., Lai, C. W., Muegge, B. D., Barisas, D., Leal-Ekman, J. S., Deepak, P., Ciorba, M. A., Liu, T. C., Hogan, D. A., Debbas, P., Braun, J., McGovern, D., Underhill, D. M., & Stappenbeck, T. S. 2021. *Debaryomyces* is enriched in Crohn's disease intestinal tissue and impairs healing in mice. *Science (New York, N.Y.)*, *371*, 1154–1159. https://doi.org/10.1126/science.abd0919.

Jayasudha, R., Das, T., Kalyana Chakravarthy, S., Sai Prashanthi, G., Bhargava, A., Tyagi, M., Rani, P. K., Pappuru, R. R., & Shivaji, S. 2020. Gut mycobiomes are altered in people with type 2 Diabetes Mellitus and Diabetic Retinopathy. *PloS one*, *15*, e0243077. https://doi.org/10.1371/journal.pone.0243077.

Jung, J. Y., Lee, S. H., Kim, J. M., Park, M. S., Bae, J. W., Hahn, Y., Madsen, E. L., &Jeon, C. O. 2011. Metagenomic analysis of kimchi, a traditional Korean fermented food. *Applied and environmental microbiology*, *77*: 2264–74. https://doi.org/10.1128/AEM.02157-10.

Kim, M. S., Park, E. J., Roh, S. W., and Bae, J. W. 2011. Diversity and abundance of single-stranded DNA viruses in human feces. *Appl. Environ. Microbiol.* 77, 8062–8070. doi: 10.1128/AEM.06331-11.

Kromhout, D., Menotti, A., Bloemberg, B., Aravanis, C., Blackburn, H., Buzina, R., Dontas, A. S., Fidanza, F., Giampaoli, S., & Jansen, A. 1995. Dietary saturated and trans fatty acids and cholesterol and 25-year mortality from coronary heart disease: the Seven Countries Study. *Preventive medicine*, *24*: 308–15. https://doi.org/10.1006/pmed.1995.1049.

Ma, G & Chen, Y. 2020. Polyphenol supplementation benefits human health via gut microbiota: A systematic review via meta-analysis. Journal of Functional Foods. 66. 103829. 10.1016/j.jff.2020.103829.

Madsen, L., Myrmel, L. S., Fjære, E., Liaset, B., & Kristiansen, K. 2017. Links between Dietary Protein Sources, the Gut Microbiota, and Obesity. *Frontiers in physiology*, *8*, 1047. https://doi.org/10.3389/fphys.2017.01047.

Maier, L., Pruteanu, M., Kuhn, M., Zeller, G., Telzerow, A., Anderson, E. E., Brochado, A. R., Fernandez, K. C., Dose, H., Mori, H., Patil, K. R., Bork, P., &Typas, A. 2018. Extensive impact of non-antibiotic drugs on human gut bacteria. *Nature*, *555*: 623–8. https://doi.org/10.1038/nature25979.

Minot, S., Wu, G. D., Lewis, J. D., and Bushman, F. D. 2012. Conservation of gene cassettes among diverse viruses of the human gut. *PLoS ONE* 7:e42342. doi: 10.1371/journal.pone.0042342.

Mitsou, E. K., Kakali, A., Antonopoulou, S., Mountzouris, K. C., Yannakoulia, M., Panagiotakos, D. B., & Kyriacou, A. 2017. Adherence to the Mediterranean diet is associated with the gut microbiota pattern and gastrointestinal characteristics in an adult population. *The British journal of nutrition*, *117*: 1645–55. https://doi.org/10.1017/S0007114517001593.

Modi, S. R., Lee, H. H., Spina, C. S., and Collins, J. J. 2013. Antibiotic treatment expands the resistance reservoir and ecological network of the phage metagenome. *Nature* 499, 219–222. doi: 10.1038/nature12212.

Nash, A. K., Auchtung, T. A., Wong, M. C., Smith, D. P., Gesell, J. R., Ross, M. C., Stewart, C. J., Metcalf, G. A., Muzny, D. M., Gibbs, R. A., Ajami, N. J., & Petrosino, J. F. 2017. The gut mycobiome of the Human Microbiome Project healthy cohort. *Microbiome*, 5, 153. https://doi.org/10.1186/s40168-017-0373-4.

Ojo, O., Feng, Q. Q., Ojo, O. O., & Wang, X. H. 2020. The Role of Dietary Fibre in Modulating Gut Microbiota Dysbiosis in Patients with Type 2 Diabetes: A Systematic Review and Meta-Analysis of Randomised Controlled Trials. *Nutrients*, 12, 3239. https://doi.org/10.3390/nu12113239.

Qin, J., Li, R., Raes, J., Arumugam, M., Burgdorf, K. S., Manichanh, C., Nielsen, T., Pons, N., Levenez, F., Yamada, T., Mende, D. R., Li, J., Xu, J., Li, S., Li, D., Cao, J., Wang, B., Liang, H., Zheng, H., Xie, Y., Wang, J. 2010. A human gut microbial gene catalogue established by metagenomic sequencing. *Nature*, 464, 59–65. https://doi.org/10.1038/nature08821.

Rasmussen, T. S., Mentzel, C. M. J., Kot, W., Castro-Mejía, J. L., Zuffa, S., Swann, J. R., Hansen, L. H., Vogensen, F. K., Hansen, A. K., Nielsen, D. S. 2020. Faecal virome transplantation decreases symptoms of type 2 diabetes and obesity in a murine model. *Gut*; 69:2122-2130.

Reyes, A., Haynes, M., Hanson, N., Angly, F. E., Heath, A. C., Rohwer, F., Gordon, J. I. 2010. Viruses in the faecal microbiota of monozygotic twins and their mothers. *Nature*, 466, 334–338. doi: 10.1038/nature09199.

Rogers, M., & Aronoff, D. M. 2016. The influence of non-steroidal anti-inflammatory drugs on the gut microbiome. *Clinical microbiology and infection : the official publication of the European Society of Clinical Microbiology and Infectious Diseases*, 22: 178.e1–178.e9. https://doi.org/10.1016/j.cmi.2015.10.003.

Rutayisire, E., Huang, K., Liu, Y., & Tao, F. 2016. The mode of delivery affects the diversity and colonization pattern of the gut microbiota during the first year of infants' life: a systematic review. *BMC gastroenterology*, 16: 86. https://doi.org/10.1186/s12876-016-0498-0.

Simpson, H. L., & Campbell, B. J. 2015. Review article: dietary fibre-microbiota interactions. *Alimentary pharmacology & therapeutics*, 42, 158–179. https://doi.org/10.1111/apt.13248.

Shin, J. H., Jung, S., Kim, S. A., Kang, M. S., Kim, M. S., Joung, H., Hwang, G. S., & Shin, D. M. 2019. Differential Effects of Typical Korean Versus American-Style Diets on Gut Microbial Composition and Metabolic Profile in Healthy Overweight Koreans: A Randomized Crossover Trial. *Nutrients*, 11: 2450. https://doi.org/10.3390/nu11102450.

Smits, S. A., Leach, J., Sonnenburg, E. D., Gonzalez, C. G., Lichtman, J. S., Reid, G., Knight, R., Manjurano, A., Changalucha, J., Elias, J. E., Dominguez-Bello, M. G., & Sonnenburg, J. L. 2017. Seasonal cycling in the gut microbiome of the Hadza hunter-gatherers of Tanzania. *Science (New York, N.Y.)*, 357: 802–6. https://doi.org/10.1126/science.aan4834.

Wastyk, H. C., Fragiadakis, G. K., Perelman, D., Dahan, D., Merrill, B. D., Yu, F. B., Topf, M., Gonzalez, C. G., Van Treuren, W., Han, S., Robinson, J. L., Elias, J. E., Sonnenburg, E. D., Gardner, C. D., & Sonnenburg, J. L. 2021. Gut-microbiota-targeted diets modulate human immune status. *Cell,* 184,4137–4153.e14. https://doi.org/10.1016/j.cell.2021.06.019.

Wu, G. D., Chen, J., Hoffmann, C., Bittinger, K., Chen, Y. Y., Keilbaugh, S. A., Bewtra M, Knights D, Walters WA, Knight R, Sinha R, Gilroy E, Gupta K, Baldassano R, Nessel L, Li H, Bushman FD, Lewis JD. 2011. Linking long-term dietary patterns with gut microbial enterotypes. *Science* 334, 105–108. doi: 10.1126/science.1208344.

Wu, H., Esteve, E, Tremaroli, V., Khan, M. T., Caesar, R., Mannerås-Holm, L., Ståhlman, M., Olsson, L. M., Serino, M., Planas-Fèlix, M., Xifra, G., Mercader, J. M., Torrents, D., Burcelin, R., Ricart, W., Perkins, R., Fernàndez-Real, J. M., &Bäckhed, F. 2017. Metformin alters the gut microbiome of individuals with treatment-naive type 2 diabetes, contributing to the therapeutic effects of the drug. *Nature medicine, 23*: 850–8. https://doi.org/10.1038/nm.4345.

Xu, C., Zhu, H., & Qiu, P. 2019. Aging progression of human gut microbiota. *BMC microbiology, 19*: 236. https://doi.org/10.1186/s12866-019-1616-2.

Yang, K., Niu, J., Zuo, T., Sun, Y., Xu, Z., Tang, W., Liu, Q., Zhang, J., Ng, E., Wong, S., Yeoh, Y. K., Chan, P., Chan, F., Miao, Y., & Ng, S. C. 2021. Alterations in the Gut Virome in Obesity and Type 2 Diabetes Mellitus. *Gastroenterology, 161*, 1257–1269.e13. https://doi.org/10.1053/j.gastro.2021.06.056.

Younge, N., McCann, J. R., Ballard, J., Plunkett, C., Akhtar, S., Araújo-Pérez, F., Murtha, A., Brandon, D., & Seed, P. C. 2019. Fetal exposure to the maternal microbiota in humans and mice. *JCI insight, 4*: e127806. https://doi.org/10.1172/jci.insight.127806.

Yu, H., Guo, Z., Shen, S., & Shan, W. 2016. Effects of taurine on gut microbiota and metabolism in mice. *Amino acids, 48*, 1601–1617. https://doi.org/10.1007/s00726-016-2219-y.

Ze, X., Duncan, S. H., Louis, P., & Flint, H. J. 2012. Ruminococcus bromii is a keystone species for the degradation of resistant starch in the human colon. *The ISME journal, 6*, 1535–1543. https://doi.org/10.1038/ismej.2012.4.

Zhang, K., Bai, P., & Deng, Z. 2022. Dose-Dependent Effect of Intake of Fermented Dairy Foods on the Risk of Diabetes: Results From a Meta-analysis. *Canadian journal of diabetes, 46*, 307–312. https://doi.org/10.1016/j.jcjd.2021.09.003.

Chapter 2

Bäckhed, F., Ding, H., Wang, T., Hooper, L. V., Koh, G. Y., Nagy, A., Semenkovich, C. F., & Gordon, J. I. 2004. The gut microbiota as an environmental factor that regulates fat storage. *Proceedings of the National Academy of Sciences of the United States of America, 101*: 15718–23. https://doi.org/10.1073/pnas.0407076101.

Chimerel, C., Emery, E., Summers, D. K., Keyser, U., Gribble, F. M., & Reimann, F. 2014. Bacterial metabolite indole modulates incretin secretion from intestinal enteroendocrine L cells. *Cell reports*, 9, 1202–1208. https://doi.org/10.1016/j.celrep.2014.10.032.

Dzidic, M., Boix-Amorós, A., Selma-Royo, M., Mira, A., &Collado, M. C. 2018. Gut Microbiota and Mucosal Immunity in the Neonate. *Medical sciences* (Basel, Switzerland), 6: 56. https://doi.org/10.3390/medsci6030056.

Galazzo, G., van Best, N., Bervoets, L., Dapaah, I. O., Savelkoul, P. H., Hornef, M.W., GI-MDH consortium, Lau, S., Hamelmann, E., &Penders, J. 2020. Development of the Microbiota and Associations With Birth Mode, Diet, and Atopic Disorders in a Longitudinal Analysis of Stool Samples, Collected From Infancy Through Early Childhood. *Gastroenterology*, 158: 1584–96. https://doi.org/10.1053/j.gastro.2020.01.024.

Hamer, H. M., Jonkers, D., Venema, K., Vanhoutvin, S., Troost, F. J., & Brummer, R. J. 2008. Review article: the role of butyrate on colonic function. *Alimentary pharmacology & therapeutics*, 27: 104–19. https://doi.org/10.1111/j.1365-2036.2007.03562.x.

Heianza, Y., Ma, W., Manson, J. E., Rexrode, K. M., & Qi, L. 2017. Gut Microbiota Metabolites and Risk of Major Adverse Cardiovascular Disease Events and Death: A Systematic Review and Meta-Analysis of Prospective Studies. *Journal of the American Heart Association*, 6, e004947. https://doi.org/10.1161/JAHA.116.004947.

Konieczna, P., Groeger, D., Ziegler, M., Frei, R., Ferstl, R., Shanahan, F., Quigley, E. M., Kiely, B., Akdis, C. A., Mahony, L. 2012. Bifidobacterium infantis 35624 administration induces Foxp3 T regulatory cells in human peripheral blood: potential role for myeloid and plasmacytoid dendritic cells. *Gut*, 61: 354–66. https://doi.org/10.1136/gutjnl-2011-300936.

Li, Z., Yi, C. X., Katiraei, S., Kooijman, S., Zhou, E., Chung, C. K., Gao, Y., van den Heuvel, J. K., Meijer, O. C., Berbée, J., Heijink, M., Giera, M., Willems van Dijk, K., Groen, A. K., Rensen, P., & Wang, Y. 2018. Butyrate reduces appetite and activates brown adipose tissue via the gut-brain neural circuit. Gut, 67: 1269–79. https://doi.org/10.1136/gutjnl-2017-314050.

Ma, L., Li, H., Hu, J., Zheng, J., Zhou, J., Botchlett, R., Matthews, D., Zeng, T., Chen, L., Xiao, X., Athrey, G., Threadgill, D. W., Li, Q., Glaser, S., Francis, H., Meng, F., Li, Q., Alpini, G., & Wu, C. 2020. Indole Alleviates Diet-Induced Hepatic Steatosis and Inflammation in a Manner Involving Myeloid Cell 6-Phosphofructo-2-Kinase/Fructose-2,6-Biphosphatase 3. *Hepatology (Baltimore, Md.)*, 72, 1191–1203. https://doi.org/10.1002/hep.31115.

Martens, E. C., Chiang, H. C., & Gordon, J. I. 2008. Mucosal glycan foraging enhances fitness and transmission of a saccharolytic human gut bacterial symbiont. Cell host & microbe, 4: 447–57. https://doi.org/10.1016/j.chom.2008.09.007.

Peng, L., Li, Z. R., Green, R. S., Holzman, I. R., & Lin, J. 2009. Butyrate enhances the intestinal barrier by facilitating tight junction assembly via activation of AMP-activated protein kinase in Caco-2 cell monolayers. *The Journal of nutrition*, 139: 1619–25. https://doi.org/10.3945/jn.109.104638.

Qiu, J., Heller, J. J., Guo, X., Chen, Z. M., Fish, K., Fu, Y. X., & Zhou, L. 2012. The aryl hydrocarbon receptor regulates gut immunity through modulation of innate lymphoid cells. *Immunity*, 36, 92–104. https://doi.org/10.1016/j.immuni.2011.11.011.

Shimada, Y., Kinoshita, M., Harada, K., Mizutani, M., Masahata, K., Kayama, H., & Takeda, K. 2013. Commensal bacteria-dependent indole production enhances epithelial barrier function in the colon. *PloS one*, 8, e80604. https://doi.org/10.1371/journal.pone.0080604.

Shimotoyodome, A., Meguro, S., Hase, T., Tokimitsu, I., & Sakata, T. 2000. Short chain fatty acids but not lactate or succinate stimulate mucus release in the rat colon. *Comparative biochemistry and physiology. Part A, Molecular & integrative physiology*, 125: 525–31. https://doi.org/10.1016/s1095-6433(00)00183-5.

Smits, H. H., Engering, A., van der Kleij, D., de Jong, E. C., Schipper, K., van Capel, T. M., Zaat, B. A., Yazdanbakhsh, M., Wierenga, E. A., van Kooyk, Y., & Kapsenberg, M. L. 2005. Selective probiotic bacteria induce IL-10-producing regulatory T cells in vitro by modulating dendritic cell function through dendritic cell- specific intercellular adhesion molecule 3-grabbing nonintegrin. *The Journal of allergy and clinical immunology*, 115:1260–67. https://doi.org/10.1016/j.jaci.2005.03.036.

Tang, W. H., Wang, Z., Levison, B. S., Koeth, R. A., Britt, E. B., Fu, X., Wu, Y., & Hazen, S. L. 2013. Intestinal microbial metabolism of phosphatidylcholine and cardiovascular risk. *The New England journal of medicine*, 368, 1575–1584. https://doi.org/10.1056/NEJMoa1109400.

Thomas, JP., Parker, A., Divekar, D., Carmen, P., Watson, A. 2018. PTU-066 The gut microbiota influences intestinal epithelial proliferative potential. *Gut*, 67:A204.

Zeng, H., & Chi, H. 2015. Metabolic control of regulatory T cell development and function. *Trends in immunology*, 36: 3–12. https://doi.org/10.1016/j.it.2014.08.003.

Chapter 3

Aksu, G., Genel, F., Koturoglu, G., Kurugol, Z. and Kutukculer, N., 2006. Serum immunoglobulin (IgG, IgM, IgA) and IgG subclass concentrations in healthy children: a study using nephelometric technique. *The Turkish Journal of Pediatrics*. 48: 19-24.

Björkstén, B., Naaber, P., Sepp, E., & Mikelsaar, M. 1999. The intestinal microflora in allergic Estonian and Swedish 2-year-old children. *Clinical and experimental allergy : journal of the British Society for Allergy and Clinical Immunology*, 29, 342–346. https://doi.org/10.1046/j.1365-2222.1999.00560.x.

Björkstén, B., Sepp, E., Julge, K., Voor, T., & Mikelsaar, M. 2001. Allergy development and the intestinal microflora during the first year of life. *The Journal of allergy and clinical immunology*, 108, 516–520. https://doi.org/10.1067/mai.2001.118130.

Bodansky, H. J., Staines, A., Stephenson, C., Haigh, D., & Cartwright, R. 1992. Evidence for an environmental effect in the aetiology of insulin dependent diabetes in a transmigratory population. *BMJ (Clinical research ed.)*, 304, 1020–1022. https://doi.org/10.1136/bmj.304.6833.1020.

Cash, H. L. and Hooper, L. V., 2005. Commensal bacteria shape intestinal immune system development. *ASM News* 71: 77-83.

Cebra, J. J., 1999. Influences of microbiota on intestinal immune system development. *American Journal of Clinical Nutrition* 69: 1046S-1051S.

Costa, D. J., Marteau, P., Amouyal, M., Poulsen, L. K., Hamelmann, E., Cazaubiel, M., Housez, B., Leuillet, S., Stavnsbjerg, M., Molimard, P., Courau, S., & Bousquet, J. 2014. Efficacy and safety of the probiotic Lactobacillus paracasei LP-33 in allergic rhinitis: a double-blind, randomized, placebo-controlled trial (GA2LEN Study). *European journal of clinical nutrition*, *68*, 602–607. https://doi.org/10.1038/ejcn.2014.13.

Darabi, B., Rahmati, S., HafeziAhmadi, M. R., Badfar, G., & Azami, M. 2019. The association between caesarean section and childhood asthma: an updated systematic review and meta-analysis. *Allergy, asthma, and clinical immunology: official journal of the Canadian Society of Allergy and Clinical Immunology*, *15*, 62. https://doi.org/10.1186/s13223-019-0367-9.

Dennis-Wall, J. C., Culpepper, T., Nieves, C., Jr, Rowe, C. C., Burns, A. M., Rusch, C. T., Federico, A., Ukhanova, M., Waugh, S., Mai, V., Christman, M. C., & Langkamp-Henken, B. 2017. Probiotics (*Lactobacillus gasseri* KS-13, *Bifidobacterium bifidum* G9-1, and *Bifidobacterium longum* MM-2) improve rhinoconjunctivitis-specific quality of life in individuals with seasonal allergies: a double-blind, placebo-controlled, randomized trial. *The American journal of clinical nutrition*, *105*, 758–767. https://doi.org/10.3945/ajcn.116.140012.

Galazzo, G., van Best, N., Bervoets, L., Dapaah, I. O., Savelkoul, P. H., Hornef, M. W., GI-MDH consortium, Lau, S., Hamelmann, E., & Penders, J. 2020. Development of the Microbiota and Associations With Birth Mode, Diet, and Atopic Disorders in a Longitudinal Analysis of Stool Samples, Collected From Infancy Through Early Childhood. *Gastroenterology*, *158*(6), 1584–1596. https://doi.org/10.1053/j.gastro.2020.01.024.

Goodman, T., & Lefrancois, L. 1989. Intraepithelial lymphocytes. Anatomical site, not T cell receptor form, dictates phenotype and function. *The Journal of experimental medicine*, *170*, 1569–1581. https://doi.org/10.1084/jem.170.5.1569.

Ismail, I. H., Oppedisano, F., Joseph, S. J., Boyle, R. J., Robins-Browne, R. M., & Tang, M. L. 2012. Prenatal administration of Lactobacillus rhamnosus has no effect on the diversity of the early infant gut microbiota. *Pediatric allergy and immunology : official publication of the European Society of Pediatric Allergy and Immunology*, *23*, 255–258. https://doi.org/10.1111/j.1399-3038.2011.01239.x.

Konieczna, P., Groeger, D., Ziegler, M., Frei, R., Ferstl, R., Shanahan, F., Quigley, E. M., Kiely, B., Akdis, C. A., & O'Mahony, L. 2012. Bifidobacterium infantis 35624 administration induces Foxp3 T regulatory cells in human peripheral blood: potential role for myeloid and plasmacytoid dendritic cells. *Gut*, *61*: 354–66. https://doi.org/10.1136/gutjnl-2011-300936.

Kukkonen, K., Savilahti, E., Haahtela, T., Juntunen-Backman, K., Korpela, R., Poussa, T., Tuure, T., & Kuitunen, M. 2007. Probiotics and prebiotic galacto-oligosaccharides in the prevention of allergic diseases: a randomized, double-blind, placebo-controlled trial. *The Journal of allergy and clinical immunology*, *119*, 192–198. https://doi.org/10.1016/j.jaci.2006.09.009.

Mowat A. M. 2003. Anatomical basis of tolerance and immunity to intestinal antigens. *Nature reviews. Immunology*, *3*, 331–341. https://doi.org/10.1038/nri1057.

Bibliography

Rutten, N. B., Gorissen, D. M., Eck, A., Niers, L. E., Vlieger, A. M., Besseling-van der Vaart, I., Budding, A. E., Savelkoul, P. H., van der Ent, C. K., & Rijkers, G. T. 2015. Long Term Development of Gut Microbiota Composition in Atopic Children: Impact of Probiotics. *PloS one*, *10*, e0137681. https://doi.org/10.1371/journal.pone.0137681.

Rowe, J., Macaubas, C., Monger, T. M., Holt, B. J., Harvey, J., Poolman, J. T., Sly, P. D. and Holt, P. G., 2000. Antigen-specific responses to diphtheria-tetanus-acellular pertussis vaccine in human infants are initially Th2 polarized. *Infection and Immunity* 68: 3873-3877.

Shroff, K. E., Meslin, K., & Cebra, J. J. 1995. Commensal enteric bacteria engender a self-limiting humoral mucosal immune response while permanently colonizing the gut. *Infection and immunity*, *63*(10), 3904–3913. https://doi.org/10.1128/iai.63.10.3904-3913.1995.

Smits, H. H., Engering, A., van der Kleij, D., de Jong, E. C., Schipper, K., van Capel, T. M., Zaat, B. A., Yazdanbakhsh, M., Wierenga, E. A., van Kooyk, Y., &Kapsenberg, M. L. 2005. Selective probiotic bacteria induce IL-10-producing regulatory T cells in vitro by modulating dendritic cell function through dendritic cell-specific intercellular adhesion molecule 3-grabbing nonintegrin. *The Journal of allergy and clinical immunology*, *115*(6):1260–67. https://doi.org/10.1016/j.jaci.2005.03.036.

Strachan D. P. 1989. Hay fever, hygiene, and household size. *BMJ (Clinical research ed.)*, *299*, 1259–1260. https://doi.org/10.1136/bmj.299.6710.1259.

Stappenbeck, T. S., Hooper, L. V., & Gordon, J. I. 2002. Developmental regulation of intestinal angiogenesis by indigenous microbes via Paneth cells. *Proceedings of the National Academy of Sciences of the United States of America*, *99*, 15451–15455. https://doi.org/10.1073/pnas.202604299.

Subbarao, P., Anand, S. S., Becker, A. B., Befus, A. D., Brauer, M., Brook, J. R., Denburg, J. A., HayGlass, K. T., Kobor, M. S., Kollmann, T. R., Kozyrskyj, A. L., Lou, W. Y., Mandhane, P. J., Miller, G. E., Moraes, T. J., Pare, P. D., Scott, J. A., Takaro, T. K., Turvey, S. E., Duncan, J. M., CHILD Study investigators 2015. The Canadian Healthy Infant Longitudinal Development (CHILD) Study: examining developmental origins of allergy and asthma. *Thorax*, *70*: 998–1000. https://doi.org/10.1136/thoraxjnl-2015-207246.

Thorburn, A. N., McKenzie, C. I., Shen, S., Stanley, D., Macia, L., Mason, L. J., Roberts, L. K., Wong, C. H., Shim, R., Robert, R., Chevalier, N., Tan, J. K., Mariño, E., Moore, R. J., Wong, L., McConville, M. J., Tull, D. L., Wood, L. G., Murphy, V. E., Mattes, J., Mackay, C. R. 2015. Evidence that asthma is a developmental origin disease influenced by maternal diet and bacterial metabolites. *Nature communications*, *6*: 7320. https://doi.org/10.1038/ncomms8320.

Wickens, K., Barthow, C., Mitchell, E. A., Stanley, T. V., Purdie, G., Rowden, J., Kang, J., Hood, F., van den Elsen, L., Forbes-Blom, E., Franklin, I., Barnes, P., Fitzharris, P., Maude, R. M., Stone, P., Abels, P., Murphy, R., & Crane, J. 2018. Maternal supplementation alone with Lactobacillus rhamnosus HN001 during pregnancy and breastfeeding does not reduce infant eczema. *Pediatric allergy and immunology : official publication of the European Society of Pediatric Allergy and Immunology*, *29*, 296–302. https://doi.org/10.1111/pai.12874.

Xu, B., Pekkanen, J., Hartikainen, A. L., & Järvelin, M. R. 2001. Caesarean section and risk of asthma and allergy in adulthood. *The Journal of allergy and clinical immunology*, *107*, 732–733. https://doi.org/10.1067/mai.2001.113048.

Zeng, H., & Chi, H. 2015. Metabolic control of regulatory T cell development and function. *Trends in immunology*, *36*: 3–12. https://doi.org/10.1016/j.it.2014.08.003.

Chapter 4

Alang, N., & Kelly, C. R. 2015. Weight gain after fecalmicrobiota transplantation. *Open forum infectious diseases*, *2*, ofv004. https://doi.org/10.1093/ofid/ofv004.

Asgharian, H., Homayouni-Rad, A., Mirghafourvand, M., & Mohammad-Alizadeh-Charandabi, S. 2020. Effect of probiotic yoghurt on plasma glucose in overweight and obese pregnant women: a randomized controlled clinical trial. *European journal of nutrition*, *59*, 205–215. https://doi.org/10.1007/s00394-019-01900-1.

Cani, P., Amar, J., Iglesias, M., Poggi, M., Knauf, C., Bastelica, D., Neyrinck, A., Fava, F., Tuohy, K., Chabo, C., Waget, A., Delmee, E., Cousin, B., Sulpice, T., Chamontin, B., Ferrieres, J., Tanti, J., Gibson, G., Casteilla, L., Delzenne, N., Alessi, M. and Burcelin, R., 2007. Metabolic Endotoxemia Initiates Obesity and Insulin Resistance. *Diabetes*, 56:1761-72.

Horvath, A., Durdevic, M., Leber, B., di Vora, K., Rainer, F., Krones, E., Douschan, P., Spindelboeck, W., Durchschein, F., Zollner, G., Stauber, R. E., Fickert, P., Stiegler, P., & Stadlbauer, V. 2020. Changes in the Intestinal Microbiome during a Multispecies Probiotic Intervention in Compensated Cirrhosis. *Nutrients*, *12*, 1874. https://doi.org/10.3390/nu12061874.

Jiao, Y., Lu, Y., & Li, X. Y. 2015. Farnesoid X receptor: a master regulator of hepatic triglyceride and glucose homeostasis. *Acta pharmacologica Sinica*, *36*, 44–50. https://doi.org/10.1038/aps.2014.116.

Kalliomäki, M., Collado, M. C., Salminen, S., & Isolauri, E. 2008. Early differences in fecal microbiota composition in children may predict overweight. *The American journal of clinical nutrition*, *87*, 534–538. https://doi.org/10.1093/ajcn/87.3.534.

Kanazawa, A., Aida, M., Yoshida, Y., Kaga, H., Katahira, T., Suzuki, L., Tamaki, S., Sato, J., Goto, H., Azuma, K., Shimizu, T., Takahashi, T., Yamashiro, Y., & Watada, H. 2021. Effects of Synbiotic Supplementation on Chronic Inflammation and the Gut Microbiota in Obese Patients with Type 2 Diabetes Mellitus: A Randomized Controlled Study. *Nutrients*, *13*, 558. https://doi.org/10.3390/nu13020558.

Karlsson, F. H., Tremaroli, V., Nookaew, I., Bergström, G., Behre, C. J., Fagerberg, B., Nielsen, J., & Bäckhed, F. 2013. Gut metagenome in European women with normal, impaired and diabetic glucose control. *Nature*, *498*, 99–103. https://doi.org/10.1038/nature12198.

Kootte, R. S., Levin, E., Salojärvi, J., Smits, L. P., Hartstra, A. V., Udayappan, S. D., Hermes, G., Bouter, K. E., Koopen, A. M., Holst, J. J., Knop, F. K., Blaak, E. E., Zhao, J., Smidt, H., Harms, A. C., Hankemeijer, T., Bergman, J., Romijn, H. A., Schaap, F. G., OldeDamink, S., Nieuwdorp, M. 2017. Improvement of Insulin Sensitivity after Lean Donor Feces in Metabolic Syndrome Is Driven by Baseline Intestinal Microbiota

Composition. *Cell metabolism*, *26*: 611–19.e6. https://doi.org/10.1016/j.cmet.2017.09.008.

Koutnikova, H., Genser, B., Monteiro-Sepulveda, M., Faurie, J. M., Rizkalla, S., Schrezenmeir, J., & Clément, K. 2019. Impact of bacterial probiotics on obesity, diabetes and non-alcoholic fatty liver disease related variables: a systematic review and meta-analysis of randomised controlled trials. *BMJ open*, *9*, e017995. https://doi.org/10.1136/bmjopen-2017-017995.

Mörkl, S., Lackner, S., Meinitzer, A., Mangge, H., Lehofer, M., Halwachs, B., Gorkiewicz, G., Kashofer, K., Painold, A., Holl, A. K., Bengesser, S. A., Müller, W., Holzer, P., & Holasek, S. J. 2018. Gut microbiota, dietary intakes and intestinal permeability reflected by serum zonulin in women. *European journal of nutrition*, *57*, 2985–2997. https://doi.org/10.1007/s00394-018-1784-0.

Perino, A., Velázquez-Villegas, L. A., Bresciani, N., Sun, Y., Huang, Q., Fénelon, V. S., Castellanos-Jankiewicz, A., Zizzari, P., Bruschetta, G., Jin, S., Baleisyte, A., Gioiello, A., Pellicciari, R., Ivanisevic, J., Schneider, B. L., Diano, S., Cota, D., & Schoonjans, K. 2021. Central anorexigenic actions of bile acids are mediated by TGR5. *Nature metabolism*, *3*, 595–603. https://doi.org/10.1038/s42255-021-00398-4.

Qin, J., Li, Y., Cai, Z., Li, S., Zhu, J., Zhang, F., Liang, S., Zhang, W., Guan, Y., Shen, D., Peng, Y., Zhang, D., Jie, Z., Wu, W., Qin, Y., Xue, W., Li, J., Han, L., Lu, D., Wu, P., Wang, J. 2012. A metagenome-wide association study of gut microbiota in type 2 diabetes. *Nature*, *490*, 55–60. https://doi.org/10.1038/nature11450.

Rondanelli, M., Miraglia, N., Putignano, P., Castagliuolo, I., Brun, P., Dall'Acqua, S., Peroni, G., Faliva, M. A., Naso, M., Nichetti, M., Infantino, V., & Perna, S. 2021. Effects of 60-Day *Saccharomyces boulardii* and Superoxide Dismutase Supplementation on Body Composition, Hunger Sensation, Pro/Antioxidant Ratio, Inflammation and Hormonal Lipo-Metabolic Biomarkers in Obese Adults: A Double-Blind, Placebo-Controlled Trial. *Nutrients*, *13*, 2512. https://doi.org/10.3390/nu13082512.

Simon, M. C., Strassburger, K., Nowotny, B., Kolb, H., Nowotny, P., Burkart, V., Zivehe, F., Hwang, J. H., Stehle, P., Pacini, G., Hartmann, B., Holst, J. J., MacKenzie, C., Bindels, L. B., Martinez, I., Walter, J., Henrich, B., Schloot, N. C., & Roden, M. 2015. Intake of Lactobacillus reuteri improves incretin and insulin secretion in glucose-tolerant humans: a proof of concept. *Diabetes care*, *38*, 1827–1834. https://doi.org/10.2337/dc14-2690.

Turnbaugh, P. J., Ley, R. E., Mahowald, M. A., Magrini, V., Mardis, E. R., & Gordon, J. I. 2006. An obesity-associated gut microbiome with increased capacity for energy harvest. *Nature*, *444*: 1027–31. https://doi.org/10.1038/nature05414.

Vrieze, A., Van Nood, E., Holleman, F., Salojärvi, J., Kootte, R. S., Bartelsman, J. F., Dallinga-Thie, G. M., Ackermans, M. T., Serlie, M. J., Oozeer, R., Derrien, M., Druesne, A., Van Hylckama Vlieg, J. E., Bloks, V. W., Groen, A. K., Heilig, H. G., Zoetendal, E. G., Stroes, E. S., de Vos, W. M., Hoekstra, J. B., Nieuwdorp, M. 2012. Transfer of intestinal microbiota from lean donors increases insulin sensitivity in individuals with metabolic syndrome. *Gastroenterology*, *143*, 913–6.e7. https://doi.org/10.1053/j.gastro.2012.06.031.

Wang, Y. D., Chen, W. D., Moore, D. D., & Huang, W. 2008. FXR: a metabolic regulator and cell protector. *Cell research*, *18*, 1087–1095. https://doi.org/10.1038/cr.2008.289.

Wu, H., Tremaroli, V., Schmidt, C., Lundqvist, A., Olsson, L. M., Krämer, M., Gummesson, A., Perkins, R., Bergström, G., & Bäckhed, F. 2020. The Gut Microbiota in Prediabetes and Diabetes: A Population-Based Cross-Sectional Study. *Cell metabolism*, *32*: 379–90.e3. https://doi.org/10.1016/j.cmet.2020.06.01.

Xie, C., Huang, W., Young, R. L., Jones, K. L., Horowitz, M., Rayner, C. K., & Wu, T. 2021. Role of Bile Acids in the Regulation of Food Intake, and Their Dysregulation in Metabolic Disease. *Nutrients*, *13*, 1104. https://doi.org/10.3390/nu13041104.

Yu, E. W., Gao, L., Stastka, P., Cheney, M. C., Mahabamunuge, J., Torres Soto, M., Ford, C. B., Bryant, J. A., Henn, M. R., & Hohmann, E. L. 2020. Fecal microbiota transplantation for the improvement of metabolism in obesity: The FMT-TRIM double-blind placebo-controlled pilot trial. *PLoS medicine*, *17*(3): e1003051. https://doi.org/10.1371/journal.pmed.1003051.

Chapter 5

Boutagy, N. E., Neilson, A. P., Osterberg, K. L., Smithson, A. T., Englund, T. R., Davy, B. M., Hulver, M. W., & Davy, K. P. 2015. Probiotic supplementation and trimethylamine-N-oxide production following a high-fat diet. *Obesity (Silver Spring, Md.)*, *23*, 2357–2363. https://doi.org/10.1002/oby.21212.

Chen, M. L., Zhu, X. H., Ran, L., Lang, H. D., Yi, L., & Mi, M. T. 2017. Trimethylamine-N-Oxide Induces Vascular Inflammation by Activating the NLRP3 Inflammasome Through the SIRT3-SOD2-mtROS Signaling Pathway. *Journal of the American Heart Association*, *6*, e006347. https://doi.org/10.1161/JAHA.117.006347.

Cyrus, T., Witztum, J. L., Rader, D. J., Tangirala, R., Fazio, S., Linton, M. F., & Funk, C. D. 1999. Disruption of the 12/15-lipoxygenase gene diminishes atherosclerosis in apo E-deficient mice. *The Journal of clinical investigation*, *103*, 1597–1604. https://doi.org/10.1172/JCI5897.

Ding, L., Chang, M., Guo, Y., Zhang, L., Xue, C., Yanagita, T., Zhang, T., & Wang, Y. 2018. Trimethylamine-N-oxide (TMAO)-induced atherosclerosis is associated with bile acid metabolism. *Lipids in health and disease*, *17*, 286. https://doi.org/10.1186/s12944-018-0939-6.

Dixon, A., Robertson, K., Yung, A., Que, M., Randall, H., Wellalagodage, D., Cox, T., Robertson, D., Chi, C., & Sun, J. 2020. Efficacy of Probiotics in Patients of Cardiovascular Disease Risk: a Systematic Review and Meta-analysis. *Current hypertension reports*, *22*, 74. https://doi.org/10.1007/s11906-020-01080-y.

Geng, J., Yang, C., Wang, B., Zhang, X., Hu, T., Gu, Y., & Li, J. 2018. Trimethylamine N-oxide promotes atherosclerosis via CD36-dependent MAPK/JNK pathway. *Biomedicine & pharmacotherapy = Biomedecine & pharmacotherapie*, *97*, 941–947. https://doi.org/10.1016/j.biopha.2017.11.016.

Heianza, Y., Ma, W., Manson, J. E., Rexrode, K. M., & Qi, L. 2017. Gut Microbiota Metabolites and Risk of Major Adverse Cardiovascular Disease Events and Death: A

Systematic Review and Meta-Analysis of Prospective Studies. *Journal of the American Heart Association*, 6, e004947. https://doi.org/10.1161/JAHA.116.004947.

Huang, L., Chambliss, K. L., Gao, X., Yuhanna, I. S., Behling-Kelly, E., Bergaya, S., Ahmed, M., Michaely, P., Luby-Phelps, K., Darehshouri, A., Xu, L., Fisher, E. A., Ge, W. P., Mineo, C., & Shaul, P. W. 2019. SR-B1 drives endothelial cell LDL transcytosis via DOCK4 to promote atherosclerosis. *Nature*, 569, 565–569. https://doi.org/10.1038/s41586-019-1140-4.

Tang, W. H., Wang, Z., Levison, B. S., Koeth, R. A., Britt, E. B., Fu, X., Wu, Y., & Hazen, S. L. 2013. Intestinal microbial metabolism of phosphatidylcholine and cardiovascular risk. *The New England journal of medicine*, 368, 1575–1584. https://doi.org/10.1056/NEJMoa1109400.

Tenore, G. C., Caruso, D., Buonomo, G., D'Avino, M., Ciampaglia, R., Maisto, M., Schisano, C., Bocchino, B., & Novellino, E. 2019. Lactofermented Annurca Apple Puree as a Functional Food Indicated for the Control of Plasma Lipid and Oxidative Amine Levels: Results from a Randomised Clinical Trial. *Nutrients*, 11, 122. https://doi.org/10.3390/nu11010122.

Van Parys, A., Karlsson, T., Vinknes, K. J., Olsen, T., Øyen, J., Dierkes, J., Nygård, O., & Lysne, V. 2021. Food Sources Contributing to Intake of Choline and Individual Choline Forms in a Norwegian Cohort of Patients With Stable Angina Pectoris. *Frontiers in nutrition*, 8, 676026. https://doi.org/10.3389/fnut.2021.676026.

Wang, Z., Klipfell, E., Bennett, B. J., Koeth, R., Levison, B. S., Dugar, B., Feldstein, A. E., Britt, E. B., Fu, X., Chung, Y. M., Wu, Y., Schauer, P., Smith, J. D., Allayee, H., Tang, W. H., DiDonato, J. A., Lusis, A. J., & Hazen, S. L. 2011. Gut flora metabolism of phosphatidylcholine promotes cardiovascular disease. *Nature*, 472, 57–63. https://doi.org/10.1038/nature09922.

Yang, S., Li, X., Yang, F., Zhao, R., Pan, X., Liang, J., Tian, L., Li, X., Liu, L., Xing, Y., & Wu, M. 2019. Gut Microbiota-Dependent Marker TMAO in Promoting Cardiovascular Disease: Inflammation Mechanism, Clinical Prognostic, and Potential as a Therapeutic Target. *Frontiers in pharmacology*, 10, 1360. https://doi.org/10.3389/fphar.2019.01360.

Zhu, W., Gregory, J. C., Org, E., Buffa, J. A., Gupta, N., Wang, Z., Li, L., Fu, X., Wu, Y., Mehrabian, M., Sartor, R. B., McIntyre, T. M., Silverstein, R. L., Tang, W., DiDonato, J. A., Brown, J. M., Lusis, A. J., & Hazen, S. L. 2016. Gut Microbial Metabolite TMAO Enhances Platelet Hyperreactivity and Thrombosis Risk. *Cell*, 165, 111–124. https://doi.org/10.1016/j.cell.2016.02.011.

Chapter 6

Bridgewater, L. C., Zhang, C., Wu, Y., Hu, W., Zhang, Q., Wang, J., Li, S., & Zhao, L. 2017. Gender-based differences in host behavior and gut microbiota composition in response to high fat diet and stress in a mouse model. *Scientific reports*, 7: 10776. https://doi.org/10.1038/s41598-017-11069-4.

Callaghan, B. L., Fields, A., Gee, D. G., Gabard-Durnam, L., Caldera, C., Humphreys, K. L., Goff, B., Flannery, J., Telzer, E. H., Shapiro, M., & Tottenham, N. 2020. Mind and gut: Associations between mood and gastrointestinal distress in children exposed to adversity. *Development and psychopathology*, *32*: 309–28. https://doi.org/10.1017/S0954579419000087.

Chu, C., Murdock, M. H., Jing, D., Won, T. H., Chung, H., Kressel, A. M., Tsaava, T., Addorisio, M. E., Putzel, G. G., Zhou, L., Bessman, N. J., Yang, R., Moriyama, S., Parkhurst, C. N., Li, A., Meyer, H. C., Teng, F., Chavan, S. S., Tracey, K. J., Regev, A., Artis, D. 2019. The microbiota regulate neuronal function and fear extinction learning. *Nature*, *574*: 543–48. https://doi.org/10.1038/s41586-019-1644-y.

Cohen Kadosh, K., Basso, M., Knytl, P., Johnstone, N., Lau, J., & Gibson, G. R. 2021. Psychobiotic interventions for anxiety in young people: a systematic review and meta-analysis, with youth consultation. *Translational psychiatry*, *11*, 352. https://doi.org/10.1038/s41398-021-01422-7.

Jiang, H., Ling, Z., Zhang, Y., Mao, H., Ma, Z., Yin, Y., Wang, W., Tang, W., Tan, Z., Shi, J., Li, L., & Ruan, B. 2015. Altered fecal microbiota composition in patients with major depressive disorder. *Brain, behavior, and immunity*, *48*: 186–94. https://doi.org/10.1016/j.bbi.2015.03.016.

Kimura, I., Inoue, D., Maeda, T., Hara, T., Ichimura, A., Miyauchi, S., Kobayashi, M., Hirasawa, A., & Tsujimoto, G. 2011. Short-chain fatty acids and ketones directly regulate sympathetic nervous system via G protein-coupled receptor 41 (GPR41). *Proceedings of the National Academy of Sciences of the United States of America*, *108*, 8030–8035. https://doi.org/10.1073/pnas.1016088108.

Kunze, W. A., Mao, Y. K., Wang, B., Huizinga, J. D., Ma, X., Forsythe, P., &Bienenstock, J. 2009. Lactobacillus reuteri enhances excitability of colonic AH neurons by inhibiting calcium-dependent potassium channel opening. *Journal of cellular and molecular medicine*, *13*, 2261–2270. https://doi.org/10.1111/j.1582-4934.2009.00686.x.

Le Morvan de Sequeira, C., Hengstberger, C., Enck, P., & Mack, I. 2022. Effect of Probiotics on Psychiatric Symptoms and Central Nervous System Functions in Human Health and Disease: A Systematic Review and Meta-Analysis. *Nutrients*, *14*, 621. https://doi.org/10.3390/nu14030621.

Lew, L. C., Hor, Y. Y., Yusoff, N., Choi, S. B., Yusoff, M., Roslan, N. S., Ahmad, A., Mohammad, J., Abdullah, M., Zakaria, N., Wahid, N., Sun, Z., Kwok, L. Y., Zhang, H., & Liong, M. T. 2019. Probiotic Lactobacillus plantarum P8 alleviated stress and anxiety while enhancing memory and cognition in stressed adults: A randomised, double-blind, placebo-controlled study. *Clinical nutrition (Edinburgh, Scotland)*, *38*, 2053–2064. https://doi.org/10.1016/j.clnu.2018.09.010.

Nikolova, V. L., Hall, M., Hall, L. J., Cleare, A. J., Stone, J. M., & Young, A. H. 2021. Perturbations in Gut Microbiota Composition in Psychiatric Disorders: A Review and Meta-analysis. *JAMA psychiatry*, *78*, 1343–1354. https://doi.org/10.1001/jamapsychiatry.2021.2573.

Nikolova, V., Zaidi, S. Y., Young, A. H., Cleare, A. J., & Stone, J. M. 2019. Gut feeling: randomized controlled trials of probiotics for the treatment of clinical depression: Systematic review and meta-analysis. *Therapeutic advances in psychopharmacology*, *9*, 2045125319859963. https://doi.org/10.1177/2045125319859963.

Nishida, K., Sawada, D., Kuwano, Y., Tanaka, H., & Rokutan, K. 2019. Health Benefits of *Lactobacillus gasseri* CP2305 Tablets in Young Adults Exposed to Chronic Stress: A Randomized, Double-Blind, Placebo-Controlled Study. *Nutrients*, *11*, 1859. https://doi.org/10.3390/nu11081859.

O'Mahony, S. M., Marchesi, J. R., Scully, P., Codling, C., Ceolho, A. M., Quigley, E. M., Cryan, J. F., & Dinan, T. G. 2009. Early life stress alters behavior, immunity, and microbiota in rats: implications for irritable bowel syndrome and psychiatric illnesses. *Biological psychiatry*, *65*: 263–67. https://doi.org/10.1016/j.biopsych.2008.06.026.

Schicho, R., Krueger, D., Zeller, F., Von Weyhern, C. W., Frieling, T., Kimura, H., Ishii, I., De Giorgio, R., Campi, B., & Schemann, M. 2006. Hydrogen sulfide is a novel prosecretory neuromodulator in the Guinea-pig and human colon. *Gastroenterology*, *131*, 1542–1552. https://doi.org/10.1053/j.gastro.2006.08.035.

Simpson, C. A., Diaz-Arteche, C., Eliby, D., Schwartz, O. S., Simmons, J. G., & Cowan, C. 2021. The gut microbiota in anxiety and depression - A systematic review. *Clinical psychology review*, *83*, 101943. https://doi.org/10.1016/j.cpr.2020.101943.

Sjögren, K., Engdahl, C., Henning, P., Lerner, U. H., Tremaroli, V., Lagerquist, M. K., Bäckhed, F., & Ohlsson, C. 2012. The gut microbiota regulates bone mass in mice. *Journal of bone and mineral research : the official journal of the American Society for Bone and Mineral Research*, *27*, 1357–1367. https://doi.org/10.1002/jbmr.1588.

Sudo, N., Chida, Y., Aiba, Y., Sonoda, J., Oyama, N., Yu, X. N., Kubo, C., & Koga, Y. 2004. Postnatal microbial colonization programs the hypothalamic-pituitary-adrenal system for stress response in mice. *The Journal of physiology*, *558*: 263–75. https://doi.org/10.1113/jphysiol.2004.063388.

Szczesniak, O., Hestad, K. A., Hanssen, J. F., & Rudi, K. 2016. Isovaleric acid in stool correlates with human depression. *Nutritional neuroscience*, *19*: 279–83. https://doi.org/10.1179/1476830515Y.0000000007.

van de Wouw, M., Boehme, M., Lyte, J. M., Wiley, N., Strain, C., O'Sullivan, O., Clarke, G., Stanton, C., Dinan, T. G., & Cryan, J. F. 2018. Short-chain fatty acids: microbial metabolites that alleviate stress-induced brain-gut axis alterations. *The Journal of physiology*, *596*: 4923–44. https://doi.org/10.1113/JP276431.

Valles-Colomer, M., Falony, G., Darzi, Y., Tigchelaar, E. F., Wang, J., Tito, R. Y., Schiweck, C., Kurilshikov, A., Joossens, M., Wijmenga, C., Claes, S., Van Oudenhove, L., Zhernakova, A., Vieira-Silva, S., & Raes, J. 2019. The neuroactive potential of the human gut microbiota in quality of life and depression. *Nature microbiology*, *4*, 623–632. https://doi.org/10.1038/s41564-018-0337-x.

Wallace, C., & Milev, R. 2017. The effects of probiotics on depressive symptoms in humans: a systematic review. *Annals of general psychiatry*, *16*: 14. https://doi.org/10.1186/s12991-017-0138-2.

Yano, J. M., Yu, K., Donaldson, G. P., Shastri, G. G., Ann, P., Ma, L., Nagler, C. R., Ismagilov, R. F., Mazmanian, S. K., & Hsiao, E. Y. 2015. Indigenous bacteria from the gut microbiota regulate host serotonin biosynthesis. *Cell*, *161*, 264–276. https://doi.org/10.1016/j.cell.2015.02.047.

Zagórska, A., Marcinkowska, M., Jamrozik, M., Wiśniowska, B., & Paśko, P. 2020. From probiotics to psychobiotics - the gut-brain axis in psychiatric disorders. *Beneficial microbes*, *11*, 717–732. https://doi.org/10.3920/BM2020.0063.

Zijlmans, M. A., Korpela, K., Riksen-Walraven, J. M., de Vos, W. M., & de Weerth, C. 2015. Maternal prenatal stress is associated with the infant intestinal microbiota. *Psychoneuroendocrinology*, *53*:233–45. https://doi.org/10.1016/j.psyneuen.2015.01.006.

Chapter 7

Adam, B., Liebregts, T., Gschossmann, J. M., Krippner, C., Scholl, F., Ruwe, M., & Holtmann, G. 2006. Severity of mucosal inflammation as a predictor for alterations of visceral sensory function in a rat model. *Pain*, *123*, 179–186. https://doi.org/10.1016/j.pain.2006.02.029.

Aroniadis, O. C., Brandt, L. J., Oneto, C., Feuerstadt, P., Sherman, A., Wolkoff, A. W., Kassam, Z., Sadovsky, R. G., Elliott, R. J., Budree, S., Kim, M., & Keller, M. J. 2019. Faecal microbiota transplantation for diarrhoea-predominant irritable bowel syndrome: a double-blind, randomised, placebo-controlled trial. *The lancet. Gastroenterology & hepatology*, *4*, 675–685. https://doi.org/10.1016/S2468-1253(19)30198-0.

Bibiloni, R., Fedorak, R. N., Tannock, G. W., Madsen, K. L., Gionchetti, P., Campieri, M., De Simone, C., & Sartor, R. B. 2005. VSL#3 probiotic-mixture induces remission in patients with active ulcerative colitis. *The American journal of gastroenterology*, *100*, 1539–1546. https://doi.org/10.1111/j.1572-0241.2005.41794.x.

Collins S. M. 2014. A role for the gut microbiota in IBS. *Nature reviews. Gastroenterology & hepatology*, *11*, 497–505. https://doi.org/10.1038/nrgastro.2014.40.

Colman, R. J., & Rubin, D. T. 2014. Fecal microbiota transplantation as therapy for inflammatory bowel disease: a systematic review and meta-analysis. *Journal of Crohn's & colitis*, *8*, 1569–1581. https://doi.org/10.1016/j.crohns.2014.08.006.

Crouzet, L., Gaultier, E., Del'Homme, C., Cartier, C., Delmas, E., Dapoigny, M., Fioramonti, J., & Bernalier-Donadille, A. 2013. The hypersensitivity to colonic distension of IBS patients can be transferred to rats through their fecal microbiota. *Neurogastroenterology and motility : the official journal of the European Gastrointestinal Motility Society*, *25*(4), e272–e282. https://doi.org/10.1111/nmo.12103.

Darfeuille-Michaud, A., & Colombel, J. F. 2008. Pathogenic Escherichia coli in inflammatory bowel diseases Proceedings of the 1st International Meeting on E. coli and IBD, June 2007, Lille, France. *Journal of Crohn's & colitis*, *2*, 255–262. https://doi.org/10.1016/j.crohns.2008.02.003.

Derwa, Y., Gracie, D. J., Hamlin, P. J., & Ford, A. C. 2017. Systematic review with meta-analysis: the efficacy of probiotics in inflammatory bowel disease. *Alimentary pharmacology & therapeutics*, *46*, 389–400. https://doi.org/10.1111/apt.14203.

El-Salhy, M., Valeur, J., Hausken, T., & Gunnar Hatlebakk, J. 2021. Changes in fecal short-chain fatty acids following fecal microbiota transplantation in patients with irritable

Bibliography

bowel syndrome. *Neurogastroenterology and motility: the official journal of the European Gastrointestinal Motility Society*, *33*, e13983. https://doi.org/10.1111/nmo.13983.

Ford, A. C., Harris, L. A., Lacy, B. E., Quigley, E., & Moayyedi, P. 2018. Systematic review with meta-analysis: the efficacy of prebiotics, probiotics, synbiotics and antibiotics in irritable bowel syndrome. *Alimentary pharmacology & therapeutics*, *48*, 1044–1060. https://doi.org/10.1111/apt.15001.

Ford, A. C., Quigley, E. M., Lacy, B. E., Lembo, A. J., Saito, Y. A., Schiller, L. R., Soffer, E. E., Spiegel, B. M., & Moayyedi, P. 2014. Efficacy of prebiotics, probiotics, and synbiotics in irritable bowel syndrome and chronic idiopathic constipation: systematic review and meta-analysis. *The American journal of gastroenterology*, *109*, 1547–1562. https://doi.org/10.1038/ajg.2014.202.

Fredericks, E., Theunissen, R., & Roux, S. 2020. Short chain fatty acids and monocarboxylate transporters in irritable bowel syndrome. *The Turkish journal of gastroenterology: the official journal of Turkish Society of Gastroenterology*, *31*, 840–847. https://doi.org/10.5152/tjg.2020.19856.

Gallagher, K., Catesson, A., Griffin, J. L., Holmes, E., & Williams, H. 2021. Metabolomic Analysis in Inflammatory Bowel Disease: A Systematic Review. *Journal of Crohn's & colitis*, *15*, 813–826. https://doi.org/10.1093/ecco-jcc/jjaa227.

Hollister, E. B., Oezguen, N., Chumpitazi, B. P., Luna, R. A., Weidler, E. M., Rubio-Gonzales, M., Dahdouli, M., Cope, J. L., Mistretta, T. A., Raza, S., Metcalf, G. A., Muzny, D. M., Gibbs, R. A., Petrosino, J. F., Heitkemper, M., Savidge, T. C., Shulman, R. J., & Versalovic, J. 2019. Leveraging Human Microbiome Features to Diagnose and Stratify Children with Irritable Bowel Syndrome. *The Journal of molecular diagnostics: JMD*, *21*, 449–461. https://doi.org/10.1016/j.jmoldx.2019.01.006.

Horvath, A., Dziechciarz, P., & Szajewska, H. 2011. Meta-analysis: Lactobacillus rhamnosus GG for abdominal pain-related functional gastrointestinal disorders in childhood. *Alimentary pharmacology & therapeutics*, *33*, 1302–1310. https://doi.org/10.1111/j.1365-2036.2011.04665.x.

Imdad, A., Nicholson, M. R., Tanner-Smith, E. E., Zackular, J. P., Gomez-Duarte, O. G., Beaulieu, D. B., & Acra, S. 2018. Fecal transplantation for treatment of inflammatory bowel disease. *The Cochrane database of systematic reviews*, *11*, CD012774. https://doi.org/10.1002/14651858.CD012774.pub2.

Johnsen, P. H., Hilpüsch, F., Cavanagh, J. P., Leikanger, I. S., Kolstad, C., Valle, P. C., & Goll, R. 2018. Faecal microbiota transplantation versus placebo for moderate-to-severe irritable bowel syndrome: a double-blind, randomised, placebo-controlled, parallel-group, single-centre trial. *The lancet. Gastroenterology & hepatology*, *3*, 17–24. https://doi.org/10.1016/S2468-1253(17)30338-2.

Limketkai, B. N., Akobeng, A. K., Gordon, M., & Adepoju, A. A. 2020. Probiotics for induction of remission in Crohn's disease. *The Cochrane database of systematic reviews*, *7*, CD006634. https://doi.org/10.1002/14651858.CD006634.pub.

Luczynski, P., Tramullas, M., Viola, M., Shanahan, F., Clarke, G., O'Mahony, S., Dinan, T. G., & Cryan, J. F. 2017. Microbiota regulates visceral pain in the mouse. *eLife*, *6*, e25887. https://doi.org/10.7554/eLife.25887.

Maharshak, N., Ringel, Y., Katibian, D., Lundqvist, A., Sartor, R. B., Carroll, I. M., & Ringel-Kulka, T. 2018. Fecal and Mucosa-Associated Intestinal Microbiota in Patients with Diarrhea-Predominant Irritable Bowel Syndrome. *Digestive diseases and sciences*, *63*, 1890–1899. https://doi.org/10.1007/s10620-018-5086-4.

Miquel, S., Martín, R., Lashermes, A., Gillet, M., Meleine, M., Gelot, A., Eschalier, A., Ardid, D., Bermúdez-Humarán, L. G., Sokol, H., Thomas, M., Theodorou, V., Langella, P., & Carvalho, F. A. 2016. Anti-nociceptive effect of Faecalibacterium prausnitzii in non-inflammatory IBS-like models. *Scientific reports*, *6*, 19399. https://doi.org/10.1038/srep19399.

Moayyedi, P., Surette, M. G., Kim, P. T., Libertucci, J., Wolfe, M., Onischi, C., Armstrong, D., Marshall, J. K., Kassam, Z., Reinisch, W., & Lee, C. H. 2015. Fecal Microbiota Transplantation Induces Remission in Patients With Active Ulcerative Colitis in a Randomized Controlled Trial. *Gastroenterology*, *149*, 102–109.e6. https://doi.org/10.1053/j.gastro.2015.04.001.

Nishida, A., Inoue, R., Inatomi, O., Bamba, S., Naito, Y., & Andoh, A. 2018. Gut microbiota in the pathogenesis of inflammatory bowel disease. *Clinical journal of gastroenterology*, *11*, 1–10. https://doi.org/10.1007/s12328-017-0813-5.

Pittayanon, R., Lau, J. T., Leontiadis, G. I., Tse, F., Yuan, Y., Surette, M., & Moayyedi, P. 2020. Differences in Gut Microbiota in Patients With vs Without Inflammatory Bowel Diseases: A Systematic Review. *Gastroenterology*, *158*, 930–946.e1. https://doi.org/10.1053/j.gastro.2019.11.294.

Nozu, T., Miyagishi, S., Nozu, R., Takakusaki, K., & Okumura, T. 2017. Lipopolysaccharide induces visceral hypersensitivity: role of interleukin-1, interleukin-6, and peripheral corticotropin-releasing factor in rats. *Journal of gastroenterology*, *52*, 72–80. https://doi.org/10.1007/s00535-016-1208-y.

O'Mahony, S. M., Felice, V. D., Nally, K., Savignac, H. M., Claesson, M. J., Scully, P., Woznicki, J., Hyland, N. P., Shanahan, F., Quigley, E. M., Marchesi, J. R., O'Toole, P. W., Dinan, T. G., & Cryan, J. F. 2014. Disturbance of the gut microbiota in early-life selectively affects visceral pain in adulthood without impacting cognitive or anxiety-related behaviors in male rats. *Neuroscience*, *277*, 885–901. https://doi.org/10.1016/j.neuroscience.2014.07.054.

Paramsothy, S., Paramsothy, R., Rubin, D. T., Kamm, M. A., Kaakoush, N. O., Mitchell, H. M., & Castaño-Rodríguez, N. 2017. Faecal Microbiota Transplantation for Inflammatory Bowel Disease: A Systematic Review and Meta-analysis. *Journal of Crohn's & colitis*, *11*, 1180–1199. https://doi.org/10.1093/ecco-jcc/jjx063.

Png, C. W., Lindén, S. K., Gilshenan, K. S., Zoetendal, E. G., McSweeney, C. S., Sly, L. I., McGuckin, M. A., & Florin, T. H. 2010. Mucolytic bacteria with increased prevalence in IBD mucosa augment in vitro utilization of mucin by other bacteria. *The American journal of gastroenterology*, *105*, 2420–2428. https://doi.org/10.1038/ajg.2010.281.

Preidis, G. A., Weizman, A. V., Kashyap, P. C., & Morgan, R. L. 2020. AGA Technical Review on the Role of Probiotics in the Management of Gastrointestinal Disorders. *Gastroenterology*, *159*, 708–738.e4. https://doi.org/10.1053/j.gastro.2020.05.060.

Raine, T., Bonovas, S., Burisch, J., Kucharzik, T., Adamina, M., Annese, V., Bachmann, O., Bettenworth, D., Chaparro, M., Czuber-Dochan, W., Eder, P., Ellul, P., Fidalgo,

C., Fiorino, G., Gionchetti, P., Gisbert, J. P., Gordon, H., Hedin, C., Holubar, S., Iacucci, M., Doherty, G. 2022. ECCO Guidelines on Therapeutics in Ulcerative Colitis: Medical Treatment. *Journal of Crohn's & colitis, 16*, 2–17. https://doi.org/10.1093/ecco-jcc/jjab178.

Ramos, G. P., & Papadakis, K. A. 2019. Mechanisms of Disease: Inflammatory Bowel Diseases. *Mayo Clinic proceedings, 94*, 155–165. https://doi.org/10.1016/j.mayocp.2018.09.013.

Ringel-Kulka, T., McRorie, J., & Ringel, Y. 2017. Multi-Center, Double-Blind, Randomized, Placebo-Controlled, Parallel-Group Study to Evaluate the Benefit of the Probiotic Bifidobacterium infantis 35624 in Non-Patients With Symptoms of Abdominal Discomfort and Bloating. *The American journal of gastroenterology, 112*, 145–151. https://doi.org/10.1038/ajg.2016.511.

Sokol, H., Landman, C., Seksik, P., Berard, L., Montil, M., Nion-Larmurier, I., Bourrier, A., Le Gall, G., Lalande, V., De Rougemont, A., Kirchgesner, J., Daguenel, A., Cachanado, M., Rousseau, A., Drouet, É., Rosenzwajg, M., Hagege, H., Dray, X., Klatzman, D., Marteau, P., Simon, T. 2020. Fecal microbiota transplantation to maintain remission in Crohn's disease: a pilot randomized controlled study. *Microbiome, 8*, 12. https://doi.org/10.1186/s40168-020-0792-5.

Sun, Q., Jia, Q., Song, L., & Duan, L. 2019. Alterations in fecal short-chain fatty acids in patients with irritable bowel syndrome: A systematic review and meta-analysis. *Medicine, 98*, e14513. https://doi.org/10.1097/MD.0000000000014513.

Vasant, D. H., Paine, P. A., Black, C. J., Houghton, L. A., Everitt, H. A., Corsetti, M., Agrawal, A., Aziz, I., Farmer, A. D., Eugenicos, M. P., Moss-Morris, R., Yiannakou, Y., & Ford, A. C. 2021. British Society of Gastroenterology guidelines on the management of irritable bowel syndrome. *Gut, 70*, 1214–1240. https://doi.org/10.1136/gutjnl-2021-324598.

Torres, J., Bonovas, S., Doherty, G., Kucharzik, T., Gisbert, J. P., Raine, T., Adamina, M., Armuzzi, A., Bachmann, O., Bager, P., Biancone, L., Bokemeyer, B., Bossuyt, P., Burisch, J., Collins, P., El-Hussuna, A., Ellul, P., Frei-Lanter, C., Furfaro, F., Gingert, C., Fiorino, G. 2020. ECCO Guidelines on Therapeutics in Crohn's Disease: Medical Treatment. *Journal of Crohn's & colitis, 14*, 4–22. https://doi.org/10.1093/ecco-jcc/jjz180.

Wu, J., Lv, L., & Wang, C. 2022. Efficacy of Fecal Microbiota Transplantation in Irritable Bowel Syndrome: A Meta-Analysis of Randomized Controlled Trials. *Frontiers in cellular and infection microbiology, 12*, 827395. https://doi.org/10.3389/fcimb.2022.827395.

Xu, D., Chen, V. L., Steiner, C. A., Berinstein, J. A., Eswaran, S., Waljee, A. K., Higgins, P., & Owyang, C. 2019. Efficacy of Fecal Microbiota Transplantation in Irritable Bowel Syndrome: A Systematic Review and Meta-Analysis. *The American journal of gastroenterology, 114*, 1043–1050. https://doi.org/10.14309/ajg.0000000000000198.

Yang, Z., Bu, C., Yuan, W., Shen, Z., Quan, Y., Wu, S., Zhu, C., & Wang, X. 2020. Fecal Microbiota Transplant via Endoscopic Delivering Through Small Intestine and Colon: No Difference for Crohn's Disease. *Digestive diseases and sciences, 65*, 150–157. https://doi.org/10.1007/s10620-019-05751-y.

Zhang, X. F., Guan, X. X., Tang, Y. J., Sun, J. F., Wang, X. K., Wang, W. D., & Fan, J. M. 2021. Clinical effects and gut microbiota changes of using probiotics, prebiotics or synbiotics in inflammatory bowel disease: a systematic review and meta-analysis. *European journal of nutrition*, *60*, 2855–2875. https://doi.org/10.1007/s00394-021-02503-5

Zhuang, X., Li, T., Li, M., Huang, S., Qiu, Y., Feng, R., Zhang, S., Chen, M., Xiong, L., & Zeng, Z. 2019. Systematic Review and Meta-analysis: Short-Chain Fatty Acid Characterization in Patients With Inflammatory Bowel Disease. *Inflammatory bowel diseases*, *25*, 1751–1763. https://doi.org/10.1093/ibd/izz188.

Chapter 8

Bellaiche, M., Ludwig, T., Arciszewska, M., Bongers, A., Gomes, C., Świat, A., Dakhlia, F., Piollet, A., Oozeer, R., & Vandenplas, Y. 2021. Safety and Tolerance of a Novel Anti-Regurgitation Formula: A Double-Blind, Randomized, Controlled Trial. *Journal of pediatric gastroenterology and nutrition*, *73*, 579–585. https://doi.org/10.1097/MPG.0000000000003289.

Cammarota, G., Ianiro, G., Tilg, H., Rajilić-Stojanović, M., Kump, P., Satokari, R., Sokol, H., Arkkila, P., Pintus, C., Hart, A., Segal, J., Aloi, M., Masucci, L., Molinaro, A., Scaldaferri, F., Gasbarrini, G., Lopez-Sanroman, A., Link, A., de Groot, P., de Vos, W. M., European FMT Working Group 2017. European consensus conference on faecal microbiota transplantation in clinical practice. *Gut*, *66*, 569–580. https://doi.org/10.1136/gutjnl-2016-313017.

Chang, C. J., Lin, T. L., Tsai, Y. L., Wu, T. R., Lai, W. F., Lu, C. C., & Lai, H. C. 2019. Next generation probiotics in disease amelioration. *Journal of food and drug analysis*, *27*, 615–622. https://doi.org/10.1016/j.jfda.2018.12.011.

DeFilipp, Z., Bloom, P. P., Torres Soto, M., Mansour, M. K., Sater, M., Huntley, M. H., Turbett, S., Chung, R. T., Chen, Y. B., & Hohmann, E. L. 2019. Drug-Resistant *E. coli* Bacteremia Transmitted by Fecal Microbiota Transplant. *The New England journal of medicine*, *381*, 2043–2050. https://doi.org/10.1056/NEJMoa1910437.

Eiseman, B., Silen, W., Bascom, G. S., & Kauvar, A. J. 1958. Fecal enema as an adjunct in the treatment of pseudomembranous enterocolitis. *Surgery*, *44*, 854–859.

Gibson, G. R., Hutkins, R., Sanders, M. E., Prescott, S. L., Reimer, R. A., Salminen, S. J., Scott, K., Stanton, C., Swanson, K. S., Cani, P. D., Verbeke, K., & Reid, G. 2017. Expert consensus document: The International Scientific Association for Probiotics and Prebiotics (ISAPP) consensus statement on the definition and scope of prebiotics. *Nature reviews. Gastroenterology & hepatology*, *14*, 491–502. https://doi.org/10.1038/nrgastro.2017.75.

Kao, D., Roach, B., Silva, M., Beck, P., Rioux, K., Kaplan, G. G., Chang, H. J., Coward, S., Goodman, K. J., Xu, H., Madsen, K., Mason, A., Wong, G. K., Jovel, J., Patterson, J., & Louie, T. 2017. Effect of Oral Capsule- vs Colonoscopy-Delivered Fecal Microbiota Transplantation on Recurrent Clostridium difficile Infection: A Randomized Clinical Trial. *JAMA*, *318*, 1985–1993. https://doi.org/10.1001/jama.2017.17077.

Jeong, K., Kim, M., Jeon, S. A., Kim, Y. H., & Lee, S. 2020. A randomized trial of Lactobacillus rhamnosus IDCC 3201 tyndallizate (RHT3201) for treating atopic dermatitis. *Pediatric allergy and immunology : official publication of the European Society of Pediatric Allergy and Immunology*, *31*, 783–792. https://doi.org/10.1111/pai.13269.

Kropp, C., Le Corf, K., Relizani, K., Tambosco, K., Martinez, C., Chain, F., Rawadi, G., Langella, P., Claus, S. P., & Martin, R. 2021. The Keystone commensal bacterium Christensenella minuta DSM 22607 displays anti-inflammatory properties both in vitro and in vivo. *Scientific reports*, *11*, 11494. https://doi.org/10.1038/s41598-021-90885-1.

Lee, C. H., Steiner, T., Petrof, E. O., Smieja, M., Roscoe, D., Nematallah, A., Weese, J. S., Collins, S., Moayyedi, P., Crowther, M., Ropeleski, M. J., Jayaratne, P., Higgins, D., Li, Y., Rau, N. V., & Kim, P. T. 2016. Frozen vs Fresh Fecal Microbiota Transplantation and Clinical Resolution of Diarrhea in Patients With Recurrent Clostridium difficile Infection: A Randomized Clinical Trial. *JAMA*, *315*, 142–149. https://doi.org/10.1001/jama.2015.18098.

Lin, C. W., Chen, Y. T., Ho, H. H., Kuo, Y. W., Lin, W. Y., Chen, J. F., Lin, J. H., Liu, C. R., Lin, C. H., Yeh, Y. T., Chen, C. W., Huang, Y. F., Hsu, C. H., Hsieh, P. S., & Yang, S. F. 2022. Impact of the food grade heat-killed probiotic and postbiotic oral lozenges in oral hygiene. *Aging*, *14*, 2221–2238. https://doi.org/10.18632/aging.203923.

Malagón-Rojas, J. N., Mantziari, A., Salminen, S., & Szajewska, H. 2020. Postbiotics for Preventing and Treating Common Infectious Diseases in Children: A Systematic Review. *Nutrients*, *12*, 389. https://doi.org/10.3390/nu12020389.

Plovier, H., Everard, A., Druart, C., Depommier, C., Van Hul, M., Geurts, L., Chilloux, J., Ottman, N., Duparc, T., Lichtenstein, L., Myridakis, A., Delzenne, N. M., Klievink, J., Bhattacharjee, A., van der Ark, K. C., Aalvink, S., Martinez, L. O., Dumas, M. E., Maiter, D., Loumaye, A., ... Cani, P. D. 2017. A purified membrane protein from Akkermansia muciniphila or the pasteurized bacterium improves metabolism in obese and diabetic mice. *Nature medicine*, *23*, 107–113. https://doi.org/10.1038/nm.4236.

Salminen, S., Collado, M. C., Endo, A., Hill, C., Lebeer, S., Quigley, E., Sanders, M. E., Shamir, R., Swann, J. R., Szajewska, H., & Vinderola, G. 2021. The International Scientific Association of Probiotics and Prebiotics (ISAPP) consensus statement on the definition and scope of postbiotics. *Nature reviews. Gastroenterology & hepatology*, *18*, 649–667. https://doi.org/10.1038/s41575-021-00440-6.

Xiaoya He, Shuyang Zhao, Yan Li. 2021. *Faecalibacterium prausnitzii*: A Next-Generation Probiotic in Gut Disease Improvement. *Canadian Journal of Infectious Diseases and Medical Microbiology*, vol. 2021, Article ID 6666114, 10 pages, 2021. https://doi.org/10.1155/2021/6666114.

About the Author

Ujjwal Sonika, MD, DM (AIIMS)
Associate Professor, Gastroenterology, GB Pant Hospital,
Maulana Azad Medical College, New Delhi, India
Email: usonika@gmail.com

Ujjwal Sonika is a faculty in Gastroenterology at Maulana Azad Medical College, Delhi University. He is an alumnus of All India Institute of Medical Sciences, New Delhi. He has more than 50 research publications and has authored numerous book chapters. He is a regular speaker at conferences and public lectures and is passionate about explaining complex concepts in a simple manner. This is his second book on the gut microbiome.

Index

#

16S RNA, 12
18 S rRNA, 15

A

acetate, 22, 24, 30, 31, 65, 72
Actinobacteria, 1, 2
adverse childhood experiences (ACEs), 54
Akkermansia muciniphila (*A. muciniphila*), 72, 97
allergic diseases, 24, 28, 30, 31, 32, 84
allergic disorders, ix, 5, 27, 29, 30, 31
allergic rhinitis, 31, 32, 84
alpha-diversity, 37
antibiotics, 4, 10, 14, 21, 49, 56, 60, 74, 93
antigen presenting cells (APCs), 20, 21, 28
anxiety, xi, 55, 57, 58, 90, 91, 94
asthma, 5, 24, 30, 31, 84, 85, 86
atherosclerosis, 25, 45, 46, 47, 48, 49, 88, 89

B

B cell, 28, 29
bacteriophages, 14
Bacteroides thetaiotaomicron, 18
Bacteroidetes, 1, 2, 6, 8, 18, 24, 40
beta-diversity, 37
betaine, 25, 48, 49
Bifidobacteria, 5, 6, 7, 9, 55, 56, 61, 71
Butyrate, 19, 22, 24, 38, 82

C

capsule FMT, 74
cardiovascular diseases (CVDs), xi, 25, 45, 46, 48, 49, 50
cesarean section (CS), 5, 30
cesarean-born babies, 5
Chenodeoxycholic acid (CDCA), 38
Cholic acid (CA), 38
choline, 25, 46, 48, 49, 89
chronic inflammation, 33, 52, 64, 86
chronic stress, 51, 91
clinical applications, xi, 33, 45, 51, 59
clostridium difficile infection (*C. difficile*), 4, 10, 21, 31, 41, 73, 74
complex carbohydrate(s), 2, 3, 7, 18, 22, 24, 37, 38, 64, 69, 70
cortisol, 51, 55, 56, 58

D

Debaryomyces hansenii, 15
Deoxycholic acid, 38
depression, 54, 57, 58, 90, 91
dysbiosis, 33, 34, 36, 40, 43, 49, 59, 61, 78, 80

E

early-life stress, 54, 55, 60
endotoxemia, 33, 34, 36, 39, 43, 86
enterochromaffin cells (ECs), 54
enterotypes, 9, 77, 81
epithelial tight junctions, 26
exercise, 3, 9, 11, 33, 41, 77, 78

F

Faecalibacterium prausnitzii, 40, 65, 72, 94, 97
fecal microbiota transplant (FMT), 4, 21, 41, 43, 50, 58, 63, 66, 67, 69, 70, 73, 74, 88, 92, 94, 95, 96, 97
fermented foods, 8, 69, 71, 75
Firmicutes, 1, 2, 6, 7, 8, 9, 18, 24, 40, 64, 65, 69, 72

Foxp3, 22, 24, 30, 82, 84
FXR receptor, 39

G

genetics, 5
GLP-1, 26, 39, 42
gut barrier, 17, 19, 72
gut microbiota, ix, xi, 1, 2, 3, 4, 5, 6, 7, 8, 9, 10, 11, 12, 13, 17, 18, 19, 20, 21, 22, 23, 24, 26, 27, 29, 30, 31, 32, 33, 34, 36, 37, 38, 39, 40, 41, 43, 45, 46, 48, 49, 50, 51, 52, 53, 54, 55, 56, 57, 58, 59, 60, 61, 62, 63, 64, 65, 66, 69, 70, 72, 73, 74, 77, 78,79, 80, 81, 82, 83, 84, 85, 86, 87, 88, 89, 90, 91, 92, 94, 96
gut microbiota metabolites, 17, 22, 23, 30, 53, 56, 82, 88
gut mycobiome, 15, 80
gut virome, 13, 14, 81
gut-associated lymphoid tissue (GALT), 27
gut-brain axis, 51, 52, 53, 60, 92

H

high-fat diet, 3, 4, 7, 26, 39, 47, 49, 55, 88
high-fiber diet, 7, 40, 69
Human Genome, 1, 2
Human Genome Project, 2
Hygiene hypothesis, 27, 28
Hypothalamus-pituitary-adrenal (HPA) axis, 56

I

IgA antibodies, 29
immune development, ix, 27, 53, 61
immune system, 20, 21, 27, 28, 29, 32, 64, 65, 83
immune tolerance, 29, 30
immunity, 20, 82, 84, 85, 90, 91
indole derivatives, 26
inflammatory bowel disease (IBD), 15, 19, 59, 63, 64, 65, 66, 74, 92, 93, 94, 95, 96

insulin, 7, 10, 34, 35, 36, 39, 41, 42, 43, 72, 77, 83, 86, 87
insulin receptor substrate (IRS), 35, 36
insulin resistance, 7, 34, 35, 36, 39, 41, 42, 43, 72, 86
intercellular junctions (ICJ), 19
intestinal barrier, 19, 26, 65, 82
intestinal permeability, 17, 19, 33, 34, 87
intraepithelial lymphocytes (IELs), 29
irritable bowel syndrome (IBS), 59, 60, 61, 62, 63, 70, 72, 75, 91, 92, 93, 94, 95
ITS-2 gene, 15

L

L-carnitine, 25, 46
lecithin, 25, 46
lipopolysaccharide (LPS), 2, 34, 36, 39, 61, 94
lithocholic acid, 38
low-density lipoprotein (LDL), 45, 46, 50, 89
low-grade inflammation, 19, 33, 34, 35, 39
low-grade systemic inflammation, 34

M

Malassezia, 15
M-cells, 30
Mediterranean diet, 9, 78, 79
metabolic disorders, 15, 33, 34, 39, 41, 42, 43
metabolic endotoxemia, 39, 86
metabolic syndrome, 33, 41, 72, 74, 86, 87
metabolomics, 12, 13, 17, 48, 54, 77
metagenomic analysis, 12
Methylamines, 25
microbiome, xi, xii, 1, 2, 5, 6, 7, 8, 9, 10, 11, 12, 13, 14, 17, 18, 21, 31, 32, 33, 36, 37, 40, 41, 51, 53, 54, 55, 57, 60, 63, 69, 72, 76, 77, 78, 79, 80, 81, 86, 87, 93, 95, 99
microbiome-based therapies, 69, 76
microbiome-based therapy, 63
microbiome-gut-brain axis, 53, 60

Microbiota Accessible Carbohydrates (MACs), 18, 70
microbiota therapy, 4, 43, 50, 58, 62, 63, 66, 69, 70, 71, 72, 73, 74
modifiable factors, 5, 6
mucosa-associated lymphoid tissue (MALT), 27

N

next generation probiotics (NGP), 72
next-Generation Sequencing (NGS), 12, 13
non-alcoholic fatty liver disease (NAFLD), 26, 34, 59, 87
non-steroidal anti-inflammatory drugs (NSAIDs), 11, 80

O

oxidized LDL, 46

P

Pathogen Associated Molecular Patterns (PAMPs), 20, 75
Peptide YY, 22, 24, 38, 52
Phosphatidylcholine, 48
polyphenols, 8, 70
postbiotics, 69, 70, 75, 76, 97
prebiotics, 42, 62, 69, 70, 75, 93, 96, 97
Prevotella, 2, 9, 55
probiotic supplements, 4, 71
probiotics, 31, 32, 42, 43, 49, 50, 57, 58, 62, 63, 66, 67, 69, 70, 71, 72, 74, 75, 84, 85, 87, 88, 90, 91, 92, 93, 94, 96, 97
Propionate, 24
Proteobacteria, 1, 2, 6, 65
proton-pump inhibitors (PPI), 10, 11
Psychobiotics, 72

R

recurrent *C. difficile* infection, 21, 41, 73

regulatory T cell (T-regs), 21, 30, 83, 85, 86

S

Saccharomyces, 15, 42, 87
secondary bile acids, 25, 38, 62, 66
selective serotonin reuptake inhibitors (SSRIs), 54
Serotonin, 22, 26, 54
short-chain fatty acids (SCFAs), 2, 7, 9, 22, 23, 24, 25, 30, 53, 56, 57, 62, 63, 64, 65, 69, 75, 92, 95
sleep, 10, 11, 58, 77
stress, ix, xi, 51, 54, 55, 56, 57, 58, 60, 72, 89, 90, 91, 92
stress-response, 55
symbiotic, 18

T

T-helper cells, 20
toll-like receptor (TLR) -4, 34
transcriptome, 13
trimethylamine-*N*-oxide (TMAO), 25, 45, 46, 47, 48, 49, 50, 88, 89
Tryptophan metabolites, 26
type 2 diabetes mellitus (T2DM), 34, 40, 81, 86

U

ulcerative colitis, 64, 65, 66, 67, 92, 94, 95

V

vaginal flora, 5
visceral pain, 59, 60, 93, 94
VO_2 max, 9

W

Western diet, 8